Workbook to Accompany

Fundamentals of Sectional Anatomy: An Imaging Approach

Second Edition

Denise L. Lazo, MA, RT (R) (M)
Associate Professor and Clinical Coordinator
Community College of Rhode Island
Lincoln, Rhode Island

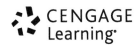
CENGAGE
Learning·

Australia • Brazil • Japan • Korea • Mexico • Singapore • Spain • United Kingdom • United States

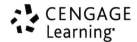

Workbook to Accompany Fundamentals of Sectional Anatomy: An Imaging Approach, Second Edition
Denise L. Lazo

Production Director: Steve Helba

Product Manager: Christina Gifford

Senior Director, Development:
Marah Bellegarde

Product Development Manager: Juliet Steiner

Senior Content Developer: Natalie Pashoukos

Product Assistant: Hannah L. Kinisky

Vice President Marketing: Jennifer Ann Baker

Marketing Director: Wendy Mapstone

Senior Production Director: Wendy A. Troeger

Production Manager: Andrew Crouth

Senior Content Project Manager:
Kara A. DiCaterino

Senior Art Director: David Arsenault

Media Editor: Debbie Bordeaux

Cover Image(s): © Cessna152/ShutterStock.com;
© Marao08/ShutterStock.com; © Allison
Herreid/ShutterStock.com

For product information and technology assistance, contact us at
Cengage Learning Customer & Sales Support, 1-800-354-9706
For permission to use material from this text or product,
submit all requests online at **www.cengage.com/permissions**
Further permissions questions can be emailed to
permissionrequest@cengage.com

ISBN-13: 978-1-133-96085-0

Cengage Learning
200 First Stamford Place
4th Floor, Stamford CT 06902
USA

Cengage Learning is a leading provider of customized learning solutions with office locations around the globe, including Singapore, the United Kingdom, Australia, Mexico, Brazil, and Japan. Locate your local office at
www.cengage.com/global

Cengage Learning products are represented in Canada by Nelson Education, Ltd.

Notice To The Reader

Printed at CLDPC, USA, 01-23

Contents

For many years, as an instructor of sectional anatomy, I was frustrated with my inability to find the perfect textbook to accompany my course. This frustration led me to write *Fundamentals of Sectional Anatomy: An Imaging Approach*. My faith in this product has been bolstered by Cengage Learning's decision to support a second edition.

For those students attempting to learn sectional anatomy, this revised workbook is a place to start testing your knowledge. Each chapter includes a variety of exercises to determine the strength of your base in sectional anatomy. A new chapter has been created, and is reflected in the newest edition of the workbook. It offers students with no preliminary background a foundation covering the anatomic position, directional terms, body planes, body cavities, body habitus, and abdominopelvic quadrants and regions. Most importantly, there are CT, and in some instances, MR images at the end of each chapter for you to test your labeling expertise. MR images have been added to Chapters 4, 6 and 7. Chapter 5 has had a section on muscles included and the exercises for that chapter register the change. The exercises on image labeling have been modified by deleting the abbreviated word lists associated with each exercise for image labeling in the first edition, replacing them with a perforated word list for each entire chapter found at the end of the book. Identify your weaknesses and refer back to the appropriate corresponding chapter in the text for clarification.

For many, if not most people repetition is a key element of learning. Presumably if you are in possession of this workbook, you are exposed to diagnostic images in a clinical setting. Complement your academic experience with mental exercises when looking at sectional images. Given the opportunity, verify your labeling with other professionals. Utilize Internet websites, entering the key words "radiographic sectional images" or some variation of this phrase. Selected sites, such as www.netanatomy.com, accessed through a subscription service at your local institution of higher learning, not only include limited series of sectional images but also incorporate the opportunity to self-test.

Good luck in your journey to becoming an expert!

Introduction

OUTLINE

EXERCISE 1-1: LABELING

Label the following illustration from the list of terms provided. (Some terms may be used more than once.)

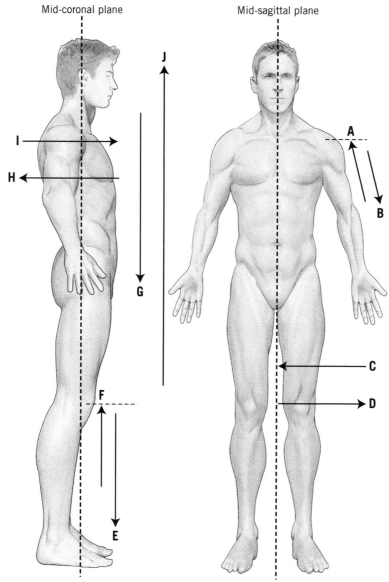

Copyright © 2015 Cengage Learning®.

caudal

cephalad

distal

dorsal

lateral

medial

proximal

ventral

A. _____

B. _____

C. _____

D. _____

E. _____

F. _____

G. _____

H. _____

I. _____

J. _____

EXERCISE 1-2: LABELING

Label the following illustration from the list of terms provided.

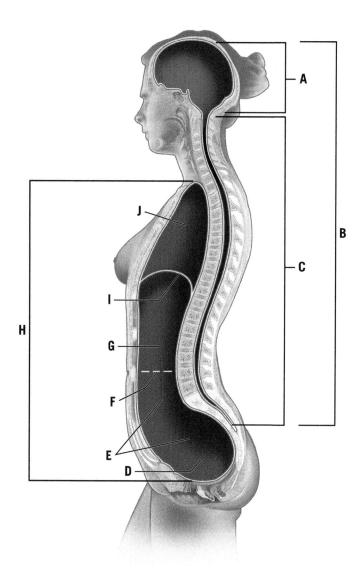

abdominal cavity

abdominopelvic cavity

cranial cavity

diaphragm

division between abdominal
and pelvic cavities

dorsal cavity

pelvic cavity

spinal cavity

thoracic cavity

ventral cavity

A. _____

B. _____

C. _____

D. _____

E. _____

F. _____

G. _____

H. _____

I. _____

J. _____

EXERCISE 1-3: LABELING

Label the following illustration from the list of terms provided.

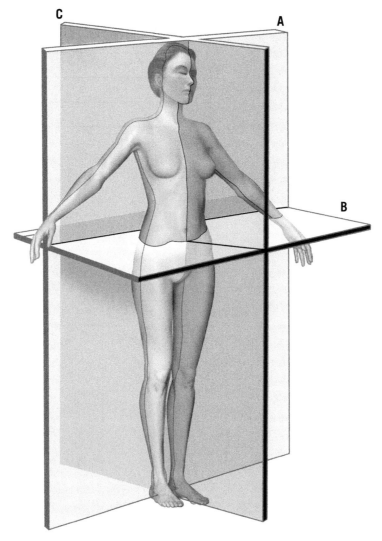

PLANES OF THE BODY

midcoronal plane
midsagittal plane
transverse plane

A. _____

B. _____

C. _____

EXERCISE 1-4: LABELING

Label the following illustration from the list of terms provided.

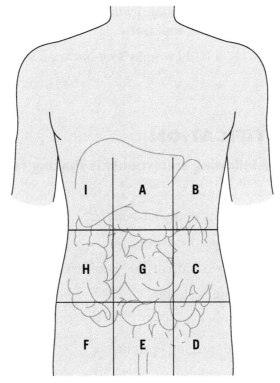

epigastric region
hypogastric region
left hypochondriac region
left inguinal region
left lumbar region
right hypochondriac region
right inguinal region
right lumbar region
umbilical region

A. _____

B. _____

C. _____

D. _____

E. _____

F. _____

G. _____

H. _____

I. _____

EXERCISE 1-5: MATCHING

Match each term with the correct description.

____ 1. asthenic

____ 2. hypersthenic

____ 3. hyposthenic

____ 4. sthenic

A. average with respect to height, weight, and torso length

B. massive, truncated build with short, broad, deep thorax

C. a slight build with long, narrow, shallow thorax, which is wider more superiorly

D. a build somewhere between asthenic and sthenic

EXERCISE 1-6: IDENTIFICATION

Indicate whether each of the following statements is making reference to (A) CT or (B) MRI.

____ 1. In general, it is better at imaging compact bone.

____ 2. It is better at demonstrating microfractures.

____ 3. Ferromagnetic objects in or near patients are problematic.

____ 4. Generally, it involves less scanning time.

____ 5. It has better tolerance for patient motion.

____ 6. It is a less expensive sectional imaging option.

____ 7. It offers better low-contrast resolution.

____ 8. Almost all images are acquired transaxially.

____ 9. Contrast media is gadolinium based.

____ 10. It relies on hydrogen atoms in the body as part of the imaging process.

____ 11. Contrast media is iodinated (ionic or nonionic) or barium sulfate.

____ 12. Images are "weighted" by PD (proton density), T1 relaxation times, or T2 relaxation times.

____ 13. The ALARA (as low as reasonably achievable) concept is promoted.

Head

OUTLINE

EXERCISE 2-1: MATCHING

Match the following terms with the correct definition.

---- 1. basal ganglia

---- 2. circle of Willis

---- 3. corpus callosum

---- 4. corpus striatum

---- 5. diploe

---- 6. gyrus

---- 7. insula

---- 8. septum pellucidum

---- 9. tectum

---- 10. vermis

a. sheet of nervous tissue separating the two lateral ventricles

b. basal ganglia composed of caudate and lentiform nucleii

c. bridge connecting the right and left cerebellar hemispheres

d. portion of the brain composed of white matter connecting the two hemispheres of the cerebrum

e. quadrigeminal plate

f. arterial anastomosis formed by internal carotid arteries, posterior cerebral arteries, anterior cerebral arteries, posterior communicating arteries, and anterior communicating artery

g. spongy bone found between two layers of compact bone in skull

h. one of four masses of gray matter located deep in the cerebrum

i. central lobe of the cerebrum

j. convolution

EXERCISE 2-2: TERM IDENTIFICATION

Provide the correct term for the following definitions.

1. Bilateral opening from the fourth ventricle, which connects it with the subarachnoid space

   _____

2. Point of communication between lateral ventricles and the third ventricle

   _____

3. Median opening of the fourth ventricle, which drains cerebrospinal fluid into the central canal of the spinal cord and the subarachnoid space

   _____

4. Passageway connecting the third and fourth ventricles of the brain

   _____

EXERCISE 2-3: COMPLETION

**Complete the following by selecting the correct term from the list provided.
(Some terms may be used more than once.)**

basal ganglia	corpus callosum	lateral (Sylvian)	quadrigeminal plate
central	cortex	longitudinal	spinal cord
centrum semiovale	diencephalon	medulla oblongata	thalamus
cerebellum	gray	midbrain	transverse
cerebral aqueduct	hypothalamus	peduncles	vermis
cerebrum	infundibulum	pons	white

In the embryo, the brain is divided into three main components: the forebrain, midbrain, and hindbrain. The forebrain is composed of the _____ and the _____. The outermost cerebrum is the _____, made of _____ matter, and the inner cerebrum is the _____, made of _____ matter, with pockets of _____ matter.

The cerebrum is divided into two hemispheres, separated by the _____ fissure. The two hemispheres communicate through the _____. Each hemisphere has five lobes: the frontal, parietal, occipital, temporal, and central. The _____ fissure separates the frontal lobe from the parietal lobe. The _____ fissure separates the frontal, parietal, and temporal lobes, and _____ the fissure separates the cerebrum from the cerebellum.

The diencephalon is composed of the _____ and _____. The _____ forms the lateral walls of the third ventricle, while the _____ acts as an intermediary between the nervous system and endocrine system and is connected to the pituitary by the _____.

The midbrain is composed of the _____, located anteriorly, and the _____, located posteriorly. Passing through the midbrain is the _____.

The hindbrain has three components: the _____, _____, and _____. The largest of the three is the _____. It is divided into two hemispheres, with the two hemispheres communicating through the _____. The most inferior portion of the hindbrain, the _____, continues as the _____ below the level of the foramen magnum.

The brain stem is made of the _____, _____, and _____.

EXERCISE 2-4: LABELING

Label the following illustration from the list of terms provided.

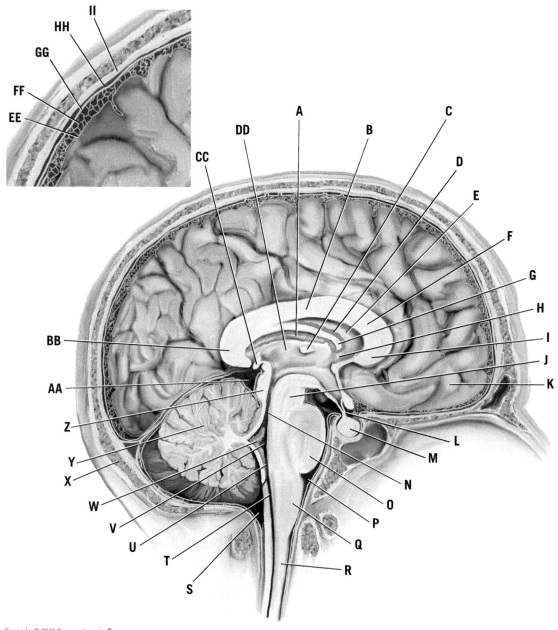

arachnoid
body of corpus callosum
central canal
cerebellum
cerebral aqueduct
cerebrum
choroid plexus of fourth ventricle
choroid plexus of lateral ventricle
choroid plexus of third ventricle
cistern pontine
cisterna magna
corpus callosum
dura mater
foramen of Magendie
foramen of Monro
fornix
fourth ventricle
genu of corpus callosum
infundibulum
intermediate mass of thalamus
lateral ventricle (anterior horn)
medulla oblongata
peduncles
pia mater
pineal gland
pituitary gland
pons
quadrigeminal cistern
quadrigeminal plate
skull
spinal cord
splenium of corpus callosum
subarachnoid space
subdural space
third ventricle

A. _____

B. _____

C. _____

D. _____

E. _____

F. _____

G. _____

H. _____

I. _____

J. _____

K. _____

L. _____

M. _____

N. _____

O. _____

P. _____

Q. _____

R. _____

S. _____

T. _____

U. _____

V. _____

W. _____

X. _____

Y. _____

Z. _____

AA. _____

BB. _____

CC. _____

DD. _____

EE. _____

FF. _____

GG. _____

HH. _____

II. _____

EXERCISE 2-5: LABELING

Label the following illustration from the list of terms provided.

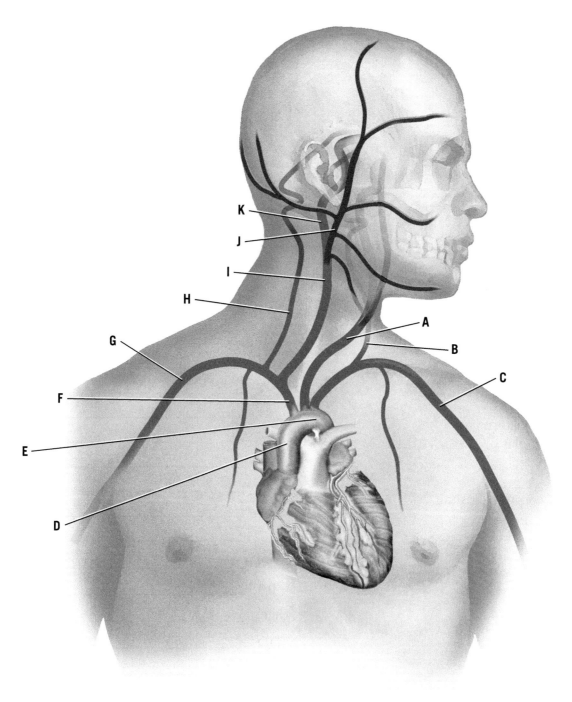

arch of aorta

ascending aorta

brachiocephalic (innominate) artery

left common carotid artery

left subclavian artery

left vertebral artery

right common carotid artery

right external carotid artery

right internal carotid artery

right subclavian artery

right vertebral artery

A. _____

B. _____

C. _____

D. _____

E. _____

F. _____

G. _____

H. _____

I. _____

J. _____

K. _____

CT AXIAL IMAGES

EXERCISE 2-6: LABELING

Label the following image from the list of terms provided in the Chapter 2 Word List in Appendix B.

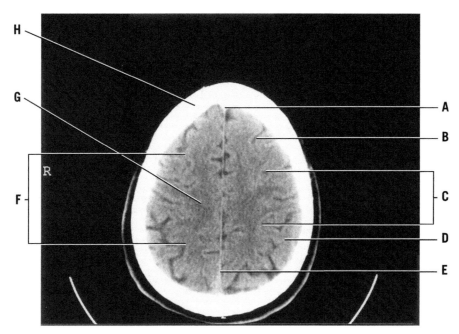

CT Images provided courtesy of Roger Williams Medical Center.

A. _____

B. _____

C. _____

D. _____

E. _____

F. _____

G. _____

H. _____

EXERCISE 2-7: LABELING

Label the following image from the list of terms provided in the Chapter 2 Word List in Appendix B.

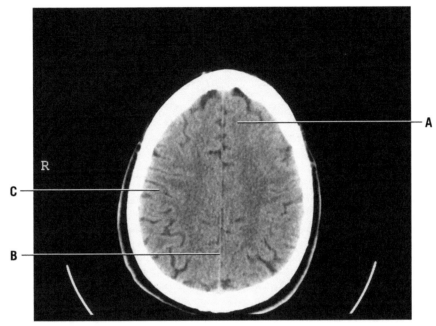

CT Images provided courtesy of Roger Williams Medical Center.

A. _____

B. _____

C. _____

EXERCISE 2-8: LABELING

Label the following image from the list of terms provided in the Chapter 2 Word List in Appendix B.

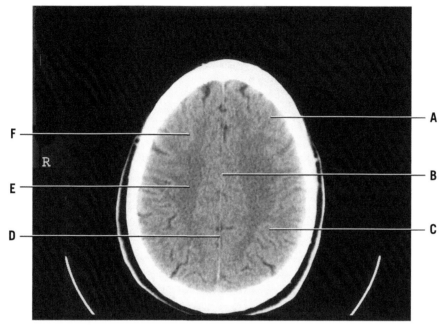

CT Images provided courtesy of Roger Williams Medical Center.

A. _____

B. _____

C. _____

D. _____

E. _____

F. _____

EXERCISE 2-9: LABELING

Label the following image from the list of terms provided in the Chapter 2 Word List in Appendix B.

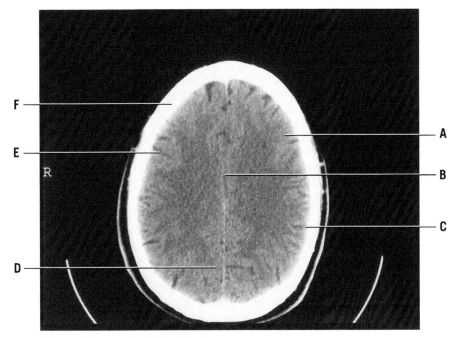

CT Images provided courtesy of Roger Williams Medical Center.

A. _____

B. _____

C. _____

D. _____

E. _____

F. _____

EXERCISE 2-10: LABELING

Label the following image from the list of terms provided in the Chapter 2 Word List in Appendix B.

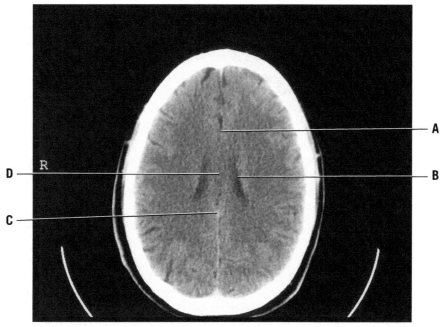

CT Images provided courtesy of Roger Williams Medical Center.

A. _____

B. _____

C. _____

D. _____

EXERCISE 2-11: LABELING

Label the following image from the list of terms provided in the Chapter 2 Word List in Appendix B.

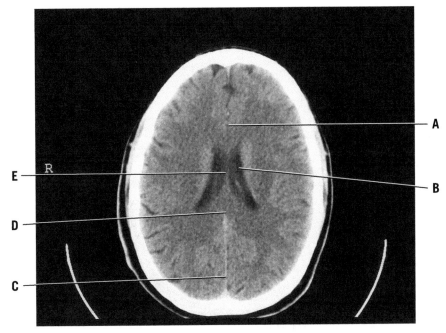

CT Images provided courtesy of Roger Williams Medical Center.

A. _____

B. _____

C. _____

D. _____

E. _____

EXERCISE 2-12: LABELING

Label the following image from the list of terms provided in the Chapter 2 Word List in Appendix B.

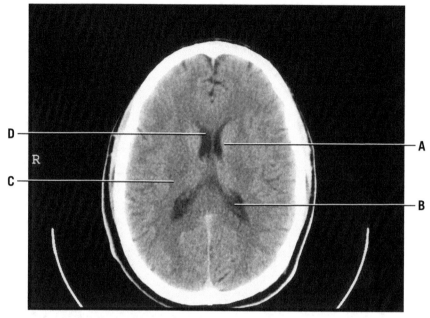

CT Images provided courtesy of Roger Williams Medical Center.

A. _____

B. _____

C. _____

D. _____

EXERCISE 2-13: LABELING

Label the following image from the list of terms provided in the Chapter 2 Word List in Appendix B.

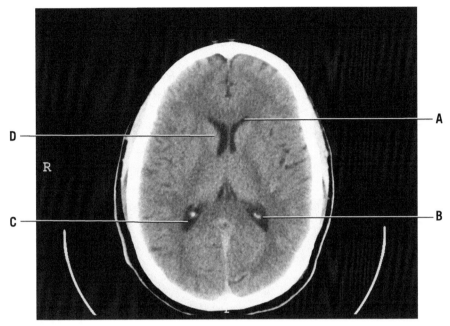

CT Images provided courtesy of Roger Williams Medical Center.

A. _____

B. _____

C. _____

D. _____

EXERCISE 2-14: LABELING

Label the following image from the list of terms provided in the Chapter 2 Word List in Appendix B.

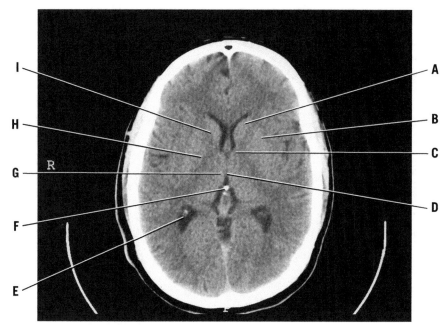

CT Images provided courtesy of Roger Williams Medical Center.

A. _____

B. _____

C. _____

D. _____

E. _____

F. _____

G. _____

H. _____

I. _____

EXERCISE 2-15: LABELING

Label the following image from the list of terms provided in the Chapter 2 Word List in Appendix B.

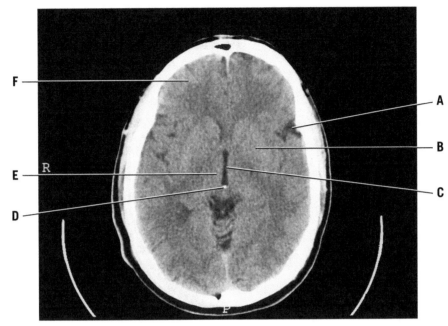

CT Images provided courtesy of Roger Williams Medical Center.

A. _____

B. _____

C. _____

D. _____

E. _____

F. _____

EXERCISE 2-16: LABELING

Label the following image from the list of terms provided in the Chapter 2 Word List in Appendix B.

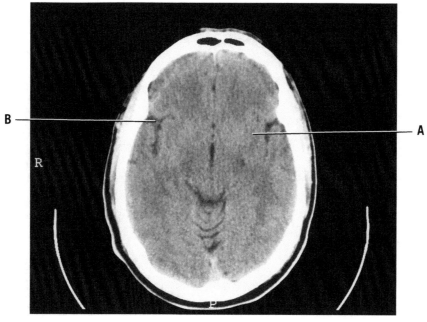

CT Images provided courtesy of Roger Williams Medical Center.

A. _____

B. _____

EXERCISE 2-17: LABELING

Label the following image from the list of terms provided in the Chapter 2 Word List in Appendix B.

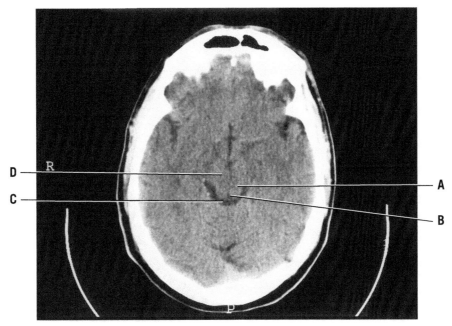

CT Images provided courtesy of Roger Williams Medical Center.

A. _____

B. _____

C. _____

D. _____

EXERCISE 2-18: LABELING

Label the following image from the list of terms provided in the Chapter 2 Word List in Appendix B.

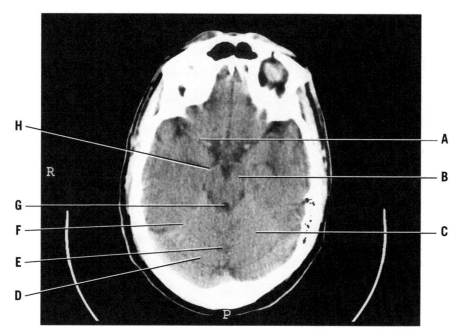

CT Images provided courtesy of Roger Williams Medical Center.

A. _____

B. _____

C. _____

D. _____

E. _____

F. _____

G. _____

H. _____

EXERCISE 2-19: LABELING

Label the following image from the list of terms provided in the Chapter 2 Word List in Appendix B.

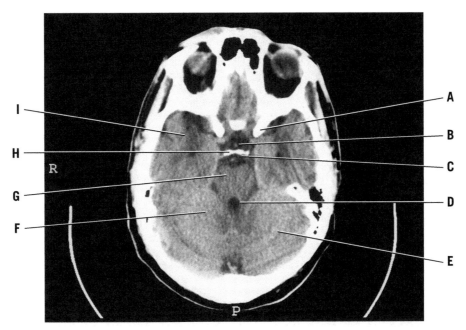

CT Images provided courtesy of Roger Williams Medical Center.

A. _____

B. _____

C. _____

D. _____

E. _____

F. _____

G. _____

H. _____

I. _____

EXERCISE 2-20: LABELING

Label the following image from the list of terms provided in the Chapter 2 Word List in Appendix B.

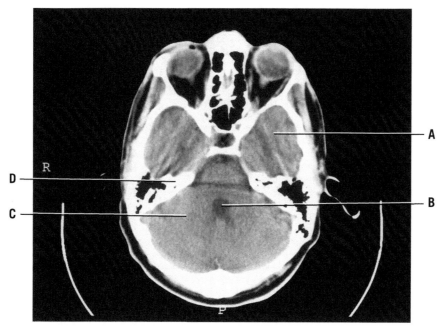

CT Images provided courtesy of Roger Williams Medical Center.

A. _____

B. _____

C. _____

D. _____

MR IMAGES

AXIAL IMAGES

EXERCISE 2-21: LABELING

Label the following image from the list of terms provided in the Chapter 2 Word List in Appendix B.

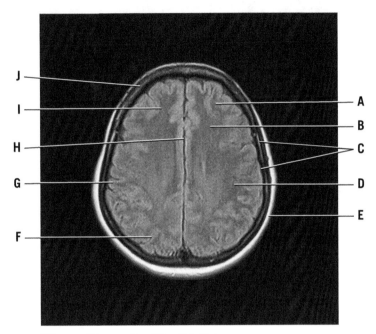

MR Images provided courtesy of Roger Williams Medical Center.

A. _____

B. _____

C. _____

D. _____

E. _____

F. _____

G. _____

H. _____

I. _____

J. _____

EXERCISE 2-22: LABELING

Label the following image from the list of terms provided in the Chapter 2 Word List in Appendix B.

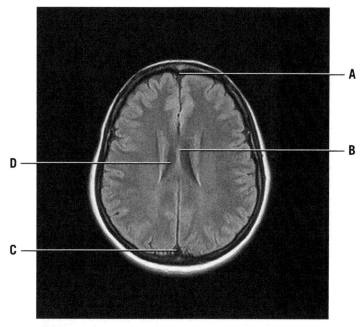

MR Images provided courtesy of Roger Williams Medical Center.

A. _____

B. _____

C. _____

D. _____

EXERCISE 2-23: LABELING

Label the following image from the list of terms provided in the Chapter 2 Word List in Appendix B.

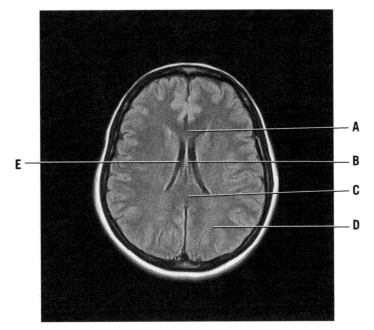

MR Images provided courtesy of Roger Williams Medical Center.

A. _____

B. _____

C. _____

D. _____

E. _____

EXERCISE 2-24: LABELING

Label the following image from the list of terms provided in the Chapter 2 Word List in Appendix B.

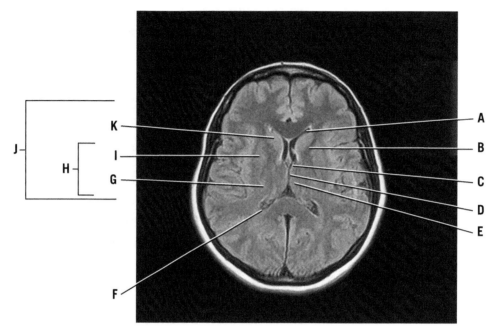

MR Images provided courtesy of Roger Williams Medical Center.

A. _____

B. _____

C. _____

D. _____

E. _____

F. _____

G. _____

H. _____

I. _____

J. _____

K. _____

EXERCISE 2-25: LABELING

Label the following image from the list of terms provided in the Chapter 2 Word List in Appendix B.

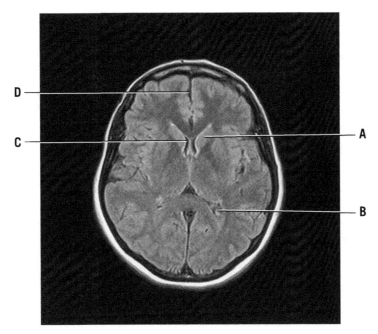

MR Images provided courtesy of Roger Williams Medical Center.

A. _____

B. _____

C. _____

D. _____

EXERCISE 2-26: LABELING

Label the following image from the list of terms provided in the Chapter 2 Word List in Appendix B.

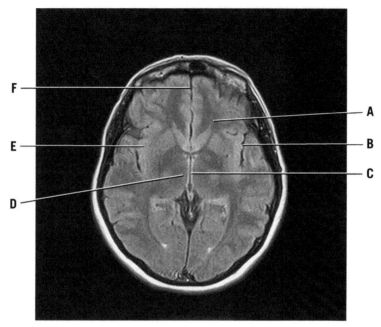

MR Images provided courtesy of Roger Williams Medical Center.

A. _____

B. _____

C. _____

D. _____

E. _____

F. _____

EXERCISE 2-27: LABELING

Label the following image from the list of terms provided in the Chapter 2 Word List in Appendix B.

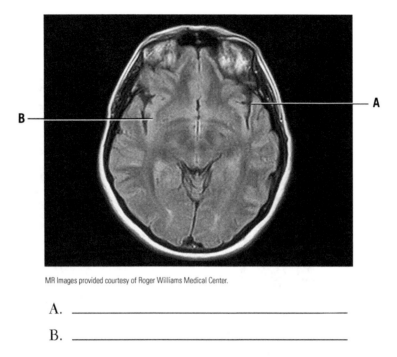

MR Images provided courtesy of Roger Williams Medical Center.

A. _____

B. _____

EXERCISE 2-28: LABELING

Label the following image from the list of terms provided in the Chapter 2 Word List in Appendix B.

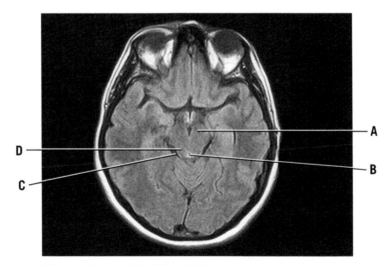

MR Images provided courtesy of Roger Williams Medical Center.

A. _____   C. _____

B. _____   D. _____

EXERCISE 2-29: LABELING

Label the following image from the list of terms provided in the Chapter 2 Word List in Appendix B.

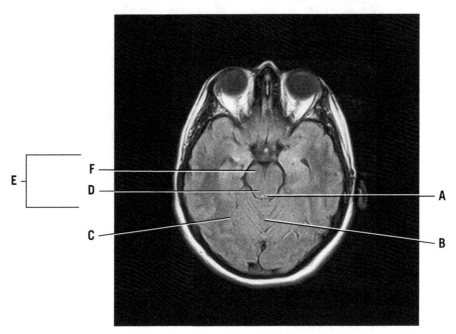

MR Images provided courtesy of Roger Williams Medical Center.

A. _____

B. _____

C. _____

D. _____

E. _____

F. _____

EXERCISE 2-30: LABELING

Label the following image from the list of terms provided in the Chapter 2 Word List in Appendix B.

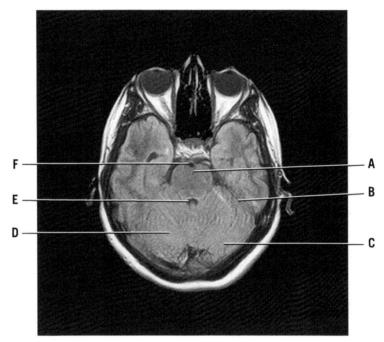

MR Images provided courtesy of Roger Williams Medical Center.

A. _____

B. _____

C. _____

D. _____

E. _____

F. _____

EXERCISE 2-31: LABELING

Label the following image from the list of terms provided in the **Chapter 2 Word List** in Appendix B.

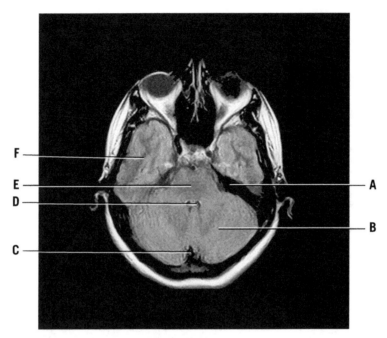

MR Images provided courtesy of Roger Williams Medical Center.

A. _____

B. _____

C. _____

D. _____

E. _____

F. _____

EXERCISE 2-32: LABELING

Label the following image from the list of terms provided in the Chapter 2 Word List in Appendix B.

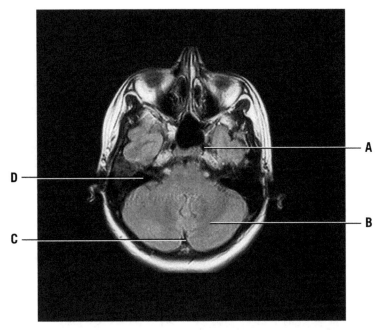

MR Images provided courtesy of Roger Williams Medical Center.

A. _____

B. _____

C. _____

D. _____

SAGITTAL IMAGE

EXERCISE 2-33: LABELING

Label the following image from the list of terms provided in the Chapter 2 Word List in Appendix B.

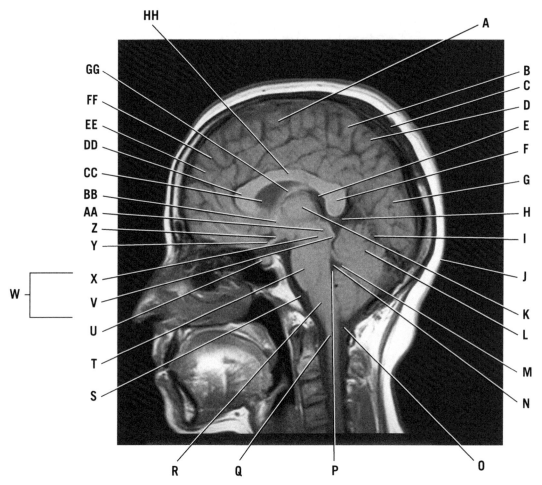

MR Images provided courtesy of Roger Williams Medical Center.

A. _____

B. _____

C. _____

D. _____

E. _____

F. _____

G. _____

H. _____

I. _____

J. _____

K. _____

L. _____

M. _____

N. _____

O. _____

P. _____

Q. _____

R. _____

S. _____

T. _____

U. _____

V. _____

W. _____

X. _____

Y. _____

Z. _____

AA. _____

BB. _____

CC. _____

DD. _____

EE. _____

FF. _____

GG. _____

HH. _____

CORONAL IMAGES

EXERCISE 2-34: LABELING

Label the following image from the list of terms provided in the Chapter 2 Word List in Appendix B.

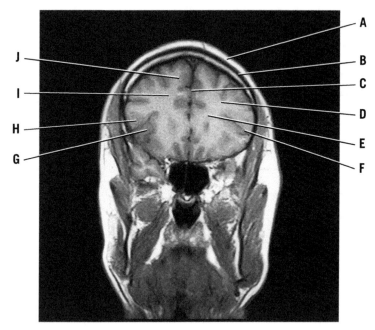

MR Images provided courtesy of Roger Williams Medical Center.

A. _____

B. _____

C. _____

D. _____

E. _____

F. _____

G. _____

H. _____

I. _____

J. _____

EXERCISE 2-35: LABELING

Label the following image from the list of terms provided in the Chapter 2 Word List in Appendix B.

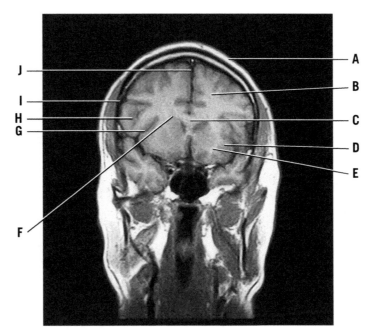

MR Images provided courtesy of Roger Williams Medical Center.

A. _____

B. _____

C. _____

D. _____

E. _____

F. _____

G. _____

H. _____

I. _____

J. _____

EXERCISE 2-36: LABELING

Label the following image from the list of terms provided in the Chapter 2 Word List in Appendix B.

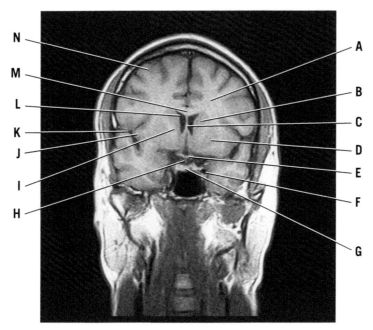

MR Images provided courtesy of Roger Williams Medical Center.

A. _____

B. _____

C. _____

D. _____

E. _____

F. _____

G. _____

H. _____

I. _____

J. _____

K. _____

L. _____

M. _____

N. _____

EXERCISE 2-37: LABELING

Label the following image from the list of terms provided in the Chapter 2 Word List in Appendix B.

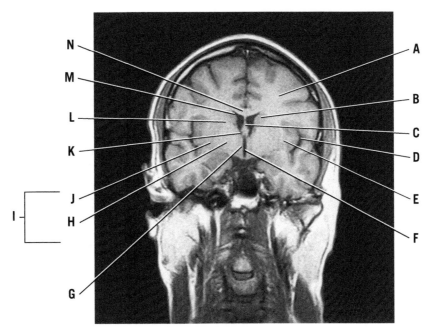

MR Images provided courtesy of Roger Williams Medical Center.

A. _____

B. _____

C. _____

D. _____

E. _____

F. _____

G. _____

H. _____

I. _____

J. _____

K. _____

L. _____

M. _____

N. _____

EXERCISE 2-38: LABELING

Label the following image from the list of terms provided in the Chapter 2 Word List in Appendix B.

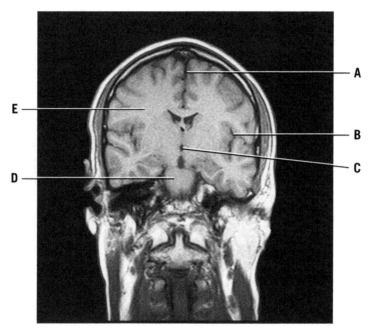

MR Images provided courtesy of Roger Williams Medical Center.

A. _____

B. _____

C. _____

D. _____

E. _____

EXERCISE 2-39: LABELING

Label the following image from the list of terms provided in the Chapter 2 Word List in Appendix B.

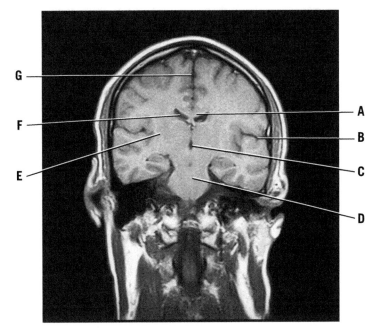

MR Images provided courtesy of Roger Williams Medical Center.

A. _____

B. _____

C. _____

D. _____

E. _____

F. _____

G. _____

EXERCISE 2-40: LABELING

Label the following image from the list of terms provided in the Chapter 2 Word List in Appendix B.

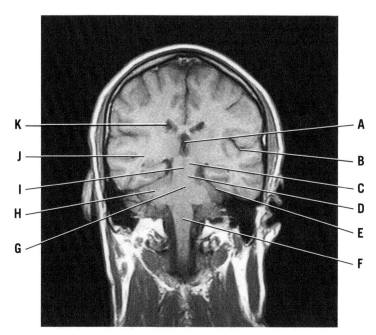

MR Images provided courtesy of Roger Williams Medical Center.

A. _____

B. _____

C. _____

D. _____

E. _____

F. _____

G. _____

H. _____

I. _____

J. _____

K. _____

EXERCISE 2-41: LABELING

Label the following image from the list of terms provided in the Chapter 2 Word List in Appendix B.

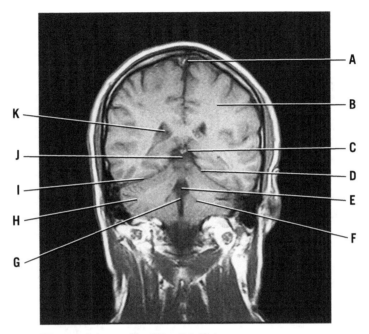

MR Images provided courtesy of Roger Williams Medical Center.

A. _____

B. _____

C. _____

D. _____

E. _____

F. _____

G. _____

H. _____

I. _____

J. _____

K. _____

EXERCISE 2-42: LABELING

Label the following image from the list of terms provided in the Chapter 2 Word List in Appendix B.

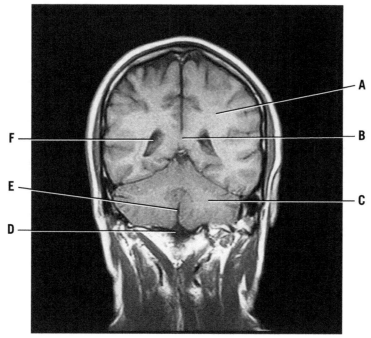

MR Images provided courtesy of Roger Williams Medical Center.

A. _____

B. _____

C. _____

D. _____

E. _____

F. _____

EXERCISE 2-43: LABELING

Label the following image from the list of terms provided in the Chapter 2 Word List in Appendix B.

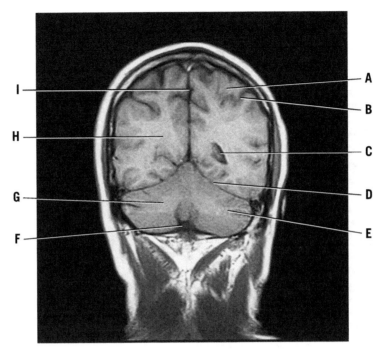

MR Images provided courtesy of Roger Williams Medical Center.

A. _____

B. _____

C. _____

D. _____

E. _____

F. _____

G. _____

H. _____

I. _____

EXERCISE 2-44: LABELING

Label the following image from the list of terms provided in the Chapter 2 Word List in Appendix B.

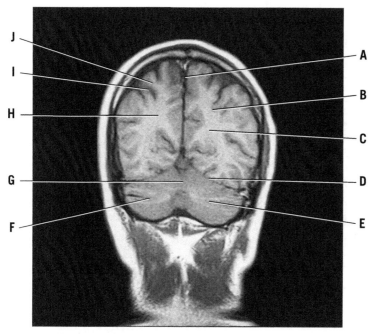

MR Images provided courtesy of Roger Williams Medical Center.

A. _____

B. _____

C. _____

D. _____

E. _____

F. _____

G. _____

H. _____

I. _____

J. _____

EXERCISE 2-45: LABELING

Label the following image from the list of terms provided in the Chapter 2 Word List in Appendix B.

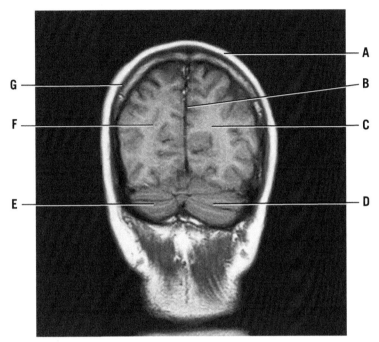

MR Images provided courtesy of Roger Williams Medical Center.

A. _____

B. _____

C. _____

D. _____

E. _____

F. _____

G. _____

EXERCISE 2-46: LABELING

Label the following image from the list of terms provided in the Chapter 2 Word List in Appendix B.

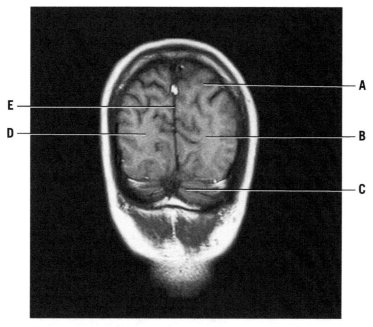

MR Images provided courtesy of Roger Williams Medical Center.

A. _____

B. _____

C. _____

D. _____

E. _____

EXERCISE 2-47: LABELING

Label the following image from the list of terms provided in the Chapter 2 Word List in Appendix B.

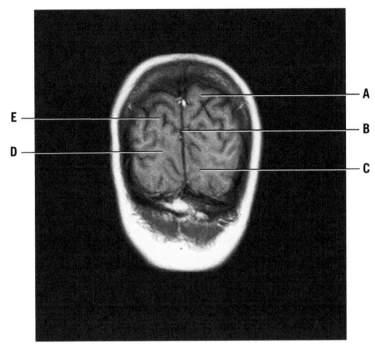

MR Images provided courtesy of Roger Williams Medical Center.

A. _____

B. _____

C. _____

D. _____

E. _____

Face

OUTLINE

EXERCISE 3-1: LABELING

Label the following illustration from the list of terms provided.

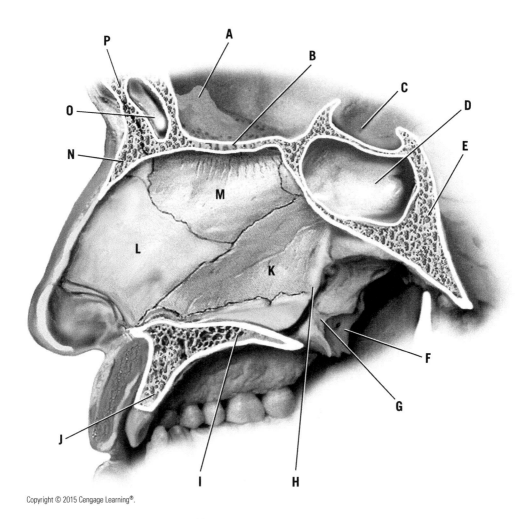

ethmoid—cribriform plate

ethmoid crista galli

ethmoid perpendicular plate

frontal bone

frontal sinus

horizontal plate of palatine bone

lateral pterygoid process of sphenoid bone

medial pterygoid process of sphenoid bone

nasal bone

palatine process of maxilla

perpendicular plate of palatine bone

septal cartilage

sphenoid bone

sphenoid sella turcica

sphenoid sinus

vomer

A. _____

B. _____

C. _____

D. _____

E. _____

F. _____

G. _____

H. _____

I. _____

J. _____

K. _____

L. _____

M. _____

N. _____

O. _____

P. _____

EXERCISE 3-2: MATCHING

Match the following terms with the correct definitions.

____ 1. alveolar process

____ 2. condyloid process

____ 3. frontal process

____ 4. palatine process

A. superior, medial extension of the maxillary bone articulating with the frontal bone

B. ridge on which the upper and lower teeth are attached on the maxillae and the mandible, respectively

C. posterior, superior portion of the mandible involved in the temporomandibular joint

D. inferior horizontal portion of the maxillary bone forming the anterior part of the roof of the mouth

EXERCISE 3-3: IDENTIFICATION

Identify the seven bones that form the orbit.

1. _____
2. _____
3. _____
4. _____
5. _____
6. _____
7. _____

EXERCISE 3-4: IDENTIFICATION

Identify the paranasal sinuses.

1. _____
2. _____
3. _____
4. _____

EXERCISE 3-5: COMPLETION

Using the list created in the previous exercise, complete the following statements.

The first paranasal sinuses to develop are the _____, and the last are the _____. The most anterior paranasal sinuses are the _____, and the most inferior are the _____. The largest paranasal sinuses are the _____.

CT CORONAL IMAGES

EXERCISE 3-6: LABELING

Label the following image from the list of terms provided in the Chapter 3 Word List in Appendix B.

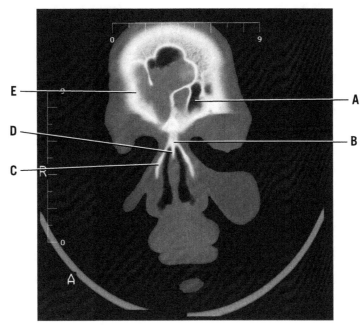

CT Images provided courtesy of Roger Williams Medical Center.

A. _____

B. _____

C. _____

D. _____

E. _____

EXERCISE 3-7: LABELING

Label the following image from the list of terms provided in the Chapter 3 Word List in Appendix B.

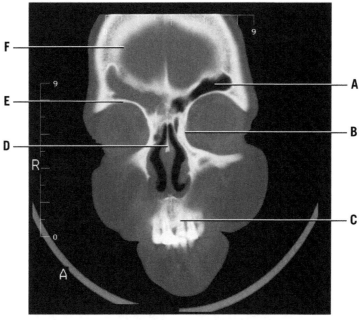

CT Images provided courtesy of Roger Williams Medical Center.

A. _____

B. _____

C. _____

D. _____

E. _____

F. _____

EXERCISE 3-8: LABELING

Label the following image from the list of terms provided in the Chapter 3 Word List in Appendix B.

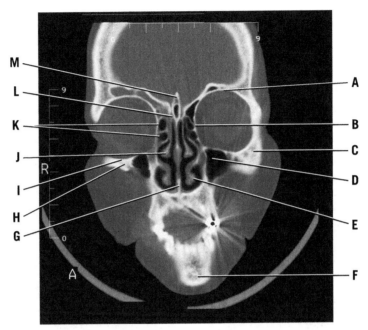

CT Images provided courtesy of Roger Williams Medical Center.

A. _____

B. _____

C. _____

D. _____

E. _____

F. _____

G. _____

H. _____

I. _____

J. _____

K. _____

L. _____

M. _____

EXERCISE 3-9: LABELING

Label the following image from the list of terms provided in the Chapter 3 Word List in Appendix B.

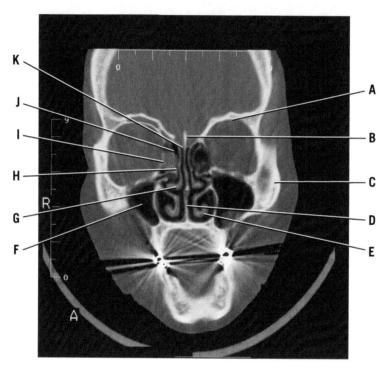

CT Images provided courtesy of Roger Williams Medical Center.

A. _____   G. _____

B. _____   H. _____

C. _____   I. _____

D. _____   J. _____

E. _____   K. _____

F. _____

EXERCISE 3-10: LABELING

Label the following image from the list of terms provided in the Chapter 3 Word List in Appendix B.

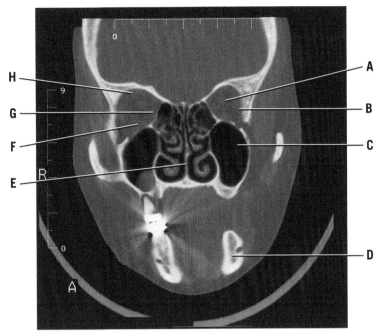

CT Images provided courtesy of Roger Williams Medical Center.

A. _____   E. _____

B. _____   F. _____

C. _____   G. _____

D. _____   H. _____

EXERCISE 3-11: LABELING

Label the following image from the list of terms provided in the Chapter 3 Word List in Appendix B.

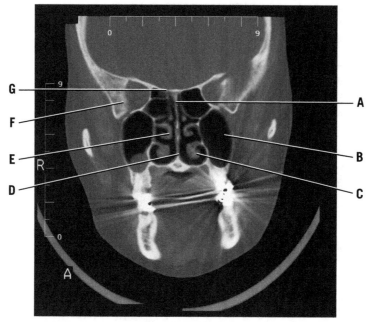

CT Images provided courtesy of Roger Williams Medical Center.

A. _____

B. _____

C. _____

D. _____

E. _____

F. _____

G. _____

EXERCISE 3-12: LABELING

Label the following image from the list of terms provided in the Chapter 3 Word List in Appendix B.

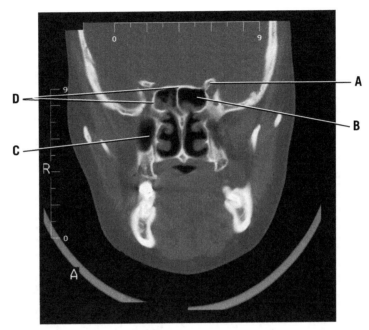

CT Images provided courtesy of Roger Williams Medical Center.

A. _____

B. _____

C. _____

D. _____

CT AXIAL IMAGES

EXERCISE 3-13: LABELING

Label the following image from the list of terms provided in the Chapter 3 Word List in Appendix B.

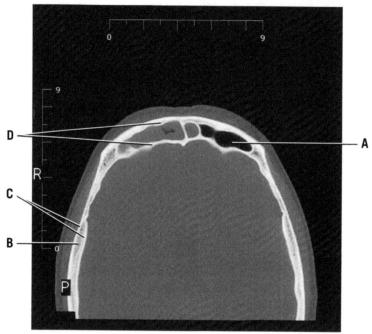

CT Images provided courtesy of Roger Williams Medical Center.

A. _____

B. _____

C. _____

D. _____

EXERCISE 3-14: LABELING

Label the following image from the list of terms provided in the Chapter 3 Word List in Appendix B.

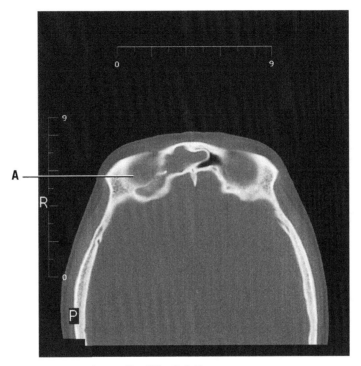

CT Images provided courtesy of Roger Williams Medical Center.

A. _____

EXERCISE 3-15: LABELING

Label the following image from the list of terms provided in the Chapter 3 Word List in Appendix B.

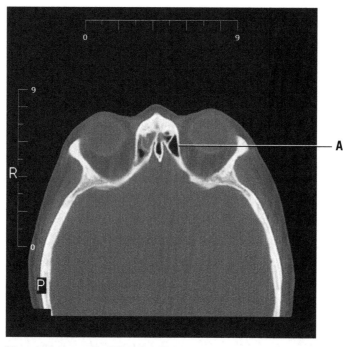

CT Images provided courtesy of Roger Williams Medical Center.

A. _____

EXERCISE 3-16: LABELING

Label the following image from the list of terms provided in the Chapter 3 Word List in Appendix B.

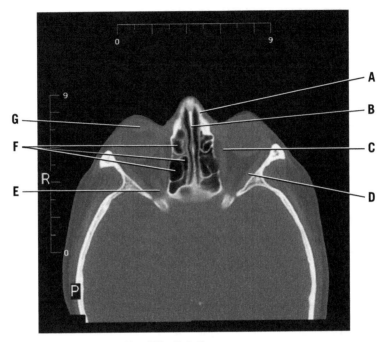

CT Images provided courtesy of Roger Williams Medical Center.

A. _____

B. _____

C. _____

D. _____

E. _____

F. _____

G. _____

EXERCISE 3-17: LABELING

Label the following image from the list of terms provided in the Chapter 3 Word List in Appendix B.

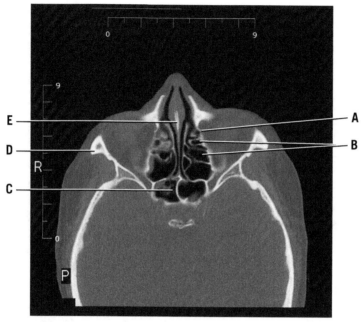

CT Images provided courtesy of Roger Williams Medical Center.

A. _____

B. _____

C. _____

D. _____

E. _____

EXERCISE 3-18: LABELING

Label the following image from the list of terms provided in the Chapter 3 Word List in Appendix B.

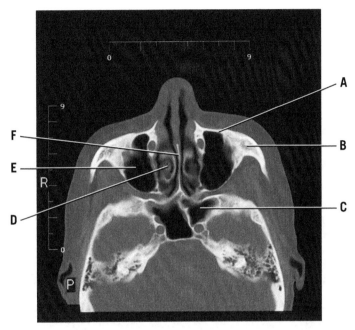

CT Images provided courtesy of Roger Williams Medical Center.

A. _____

B. _____

C. _____

D. _____

E. _____

F. _____

EXERCISE 3-19: LABELING

Label the following image from the list of terms provided in the Chapter 3 Word List in Appendix B.

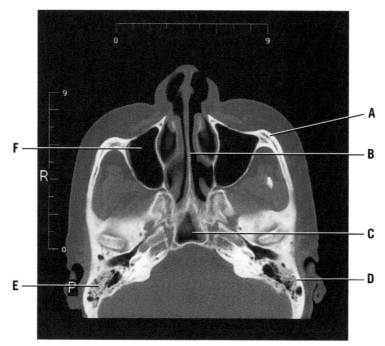

CT Images provided courtesy of Roger Williams Medical Center.

A. _____

B. _____

C. _____

D. _____

E. _____

F. _____

EXERCISE 3-20: LABELING

Label the following image from the list of terms provided in the Chapter 3 Word List in Appendix B.

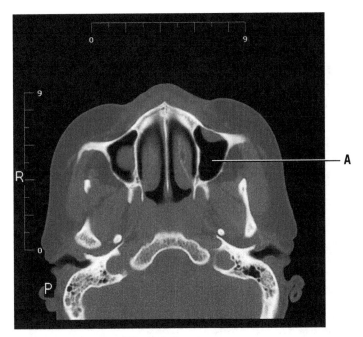

A

CT Images provided courtesy of Roger Williams Medical Center.

A. _____

EXERCISE 3-21: LABELING

Label the following image from the list of terms provided in the Chapter 3 Word List in Appendix B.

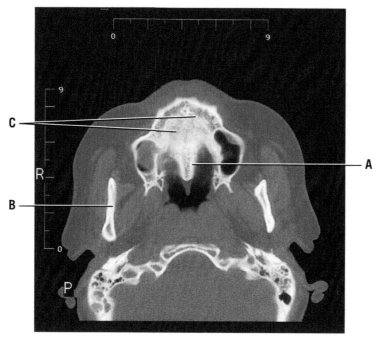

CT Images provided courtesy of Roger Williams Medical Center.

A. _____

B. _____

C. _____

EXERCISE 3-22: LABELING

Label the following image from the list of terms provided in the Chapter 3 Word List in Appendix B.

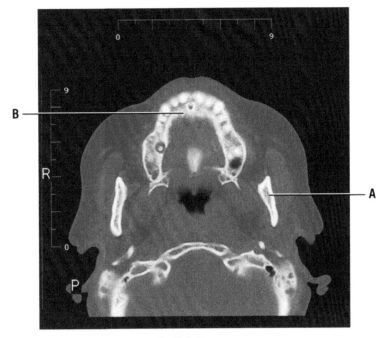

CT Images provided courtesy of Roger Williams Medical Center.

A. _____

B. _____

Neck

OUTLINE

EXERCISE 4-1: LABELING

Label the following illustration from the list of terms provided.

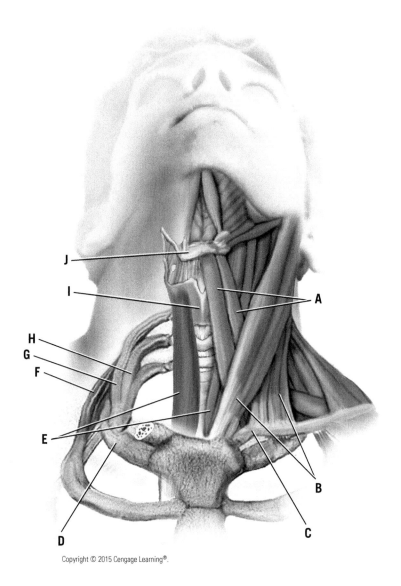

Copyright © 2015 Cengage Learning®.

anterior scalene muscle

clavicle

first rib

hyoid bone

middle scalene muscle

posterior scalene muscle

sternocleidomastoid (SCM) muscle

sternohyoid muscle

sternothyroid muscle

thyroid cartilage

A. _____

B. _____

C. _____

D. _____

E. _____

F. _____

G. _____

H. _____

I. _____

J. _____

EXERCISE 4-2: MATCHING

Match the following terms with the correct definitions.

_____ 1. corniculate

_____ 2. larynx

_____ 3. origin

_____ 4. scalene

_____ 5. sublingual

a. muscle found in the neck on either side of the cervical vertebrae

b. one of three pairs of salivary glands; found beneath the tongue

c. horn-shaped projection

d. "voice box"; surrounds the distal portion of the pharynx

e. the fixed point of attachment of a muscle

EXERCISE 4-3: IDENTIFICATION

Identify the salivary glands.

1. _____

2. _____

3. _____

EXERCISE 4-4: IDENTIFICATION

Identify the three parts of the pharynx.

1. _____

2. _____

3. _____

EXERCISE 4-5: COMPLETION

Complete the following by selecting the correct term from the list provided. (Some terms may be used more than once.)

C5/C6
cricoid cartilage
esophagus
laryngo-

right and left primary bronchi
T4/T5
trachea

The _____ pharynx bifurcates into the _____ anteriorly and the _____ posteriorly at the bottom of the _____, at approximately _____. At a lower level, the _____ bifurcates into the _____ at approximately _____. The _____ continues through the thoracic region into the abdomen.

EXERCISE 4-6: LABELING

Label the following illustration from the list of terms provided.

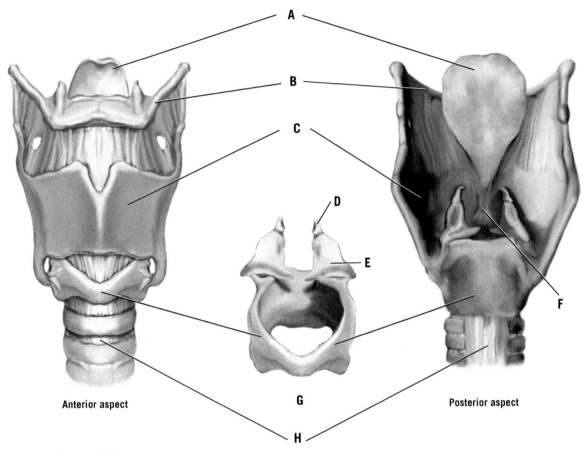

Anterior aspect

Posterior aspect

arytenoid cartilage
corniculate cartilage
cricoid cartilage
epiglottis
hyoid bone
thyroid cartilage
trachea
vocal cords

A. _____

B. _____

C. _____

D. _____

E. _____

F. _____

G. _____

H. _____

CT AXIAL IMAGES

EXERCISE 4-7: LABELING

Label the following image from the list of terms provided in the Chapter 4 Word List in Appendix B.

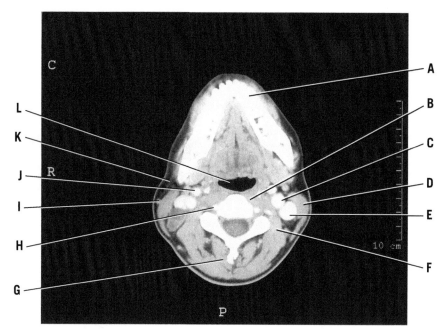

CT Images provided courtesy of Roger Williams Medical Center.

A. _____

B. _____

C. _____

D. _____

E. _____

F. _____

G. _____

H. _____

I. _____

J. _____

K. _____

L. _____

EXERCISE 4-8: LABELING

Label the following image from the list of terms provided in the Chapter 4 Word List in Appendix B.

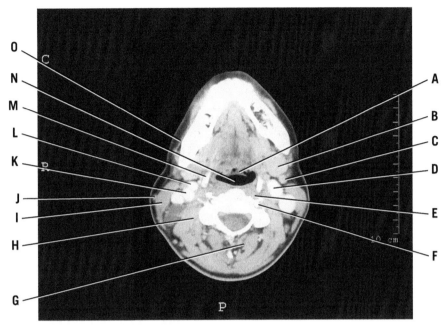

CT Images provided courtesy of Roger Williams Medical Center.

A. _____   I. _____

B. _____   J. _____

C. _____   K. _____

D. _____   L. _____

E. _____   M. _____

F. _____   N. _____

G. _____   O. _____

H. _____

EXERCISE 4-9: LABELING

Label the following image from the list of terms provided in the Chapter 4 Word List in Appendix B.

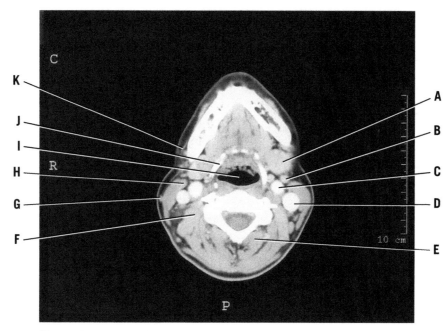

CT Images provided courtesy of Roger Williams Medical Center.

A. _____

B. _____

C. _____

D. _____

E. _____

F. _____

G. _____

H. _____

I. _____

J. _____

K. _____

EXERCISE 4-10: LABELING

Label the following image from the list of terms provided in the Chapter 4 Word List in Appendix B.

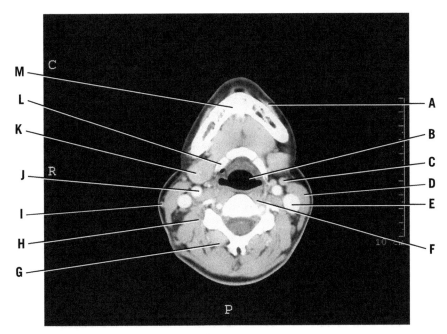

CT Images provided courtesy of Roger Williams Medical Center.

A. _____

B. _____

C. _____

D. _____

E. _____

F. _____

G. _____

H. _____

I. _____

J. _____

K. _____

L. _____

M. _____

EXERCISE 4-11: LABELING

Label the following image from the list of terms provided in the Chapter 4 Word List in Appendix B.

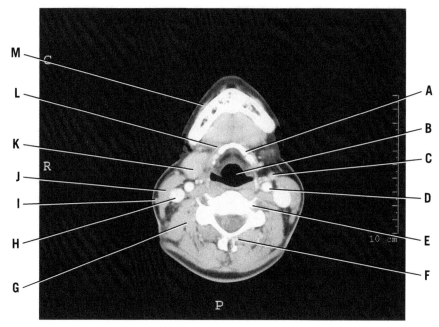

CT Images provided courtesy of Roger Williams Medical Center.

A. _____

B. _____

C. _____

D. _____

E. _____

F. _____

G. _____

H. _____

I. _____

J. _____

K. _____

L. _____

M. _____

EXERCISE 4-12: LABELING

Label the following image from the list of terms provided in the Chapter 4 Word List in Appendix B.

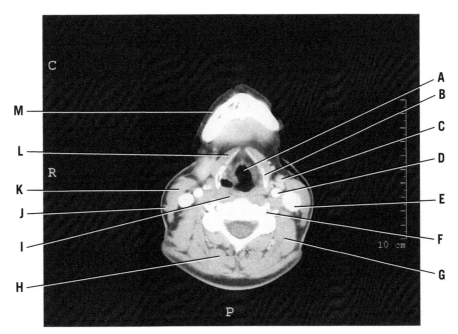

CT Images provided courtesy of Roger Williams Medical Center.

A. _____

B. _____

C. _____

D. _____

E. _____

F. _____

G. _____

H. _____

I. _____

J. _____

K. _____

L. _____

M. _____

EXERCISE 4-13: LABELING

Label the following image from the list of terms provided in the Chapter 4 Word List in Appendix B.

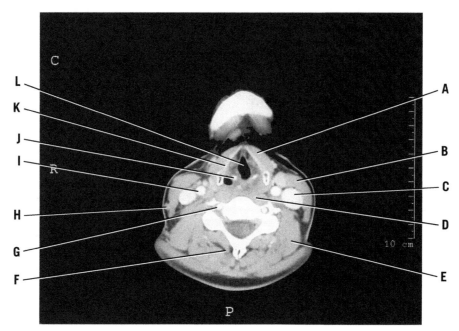

CT Images provided courtesy of Roger Williams Medical Center.

A. _____

B. _____

C. _____

D. _____

E. _____

F. _____

G. _____

H. _____

I. _____

J. _____

K. _____

L. _____

EXERCISE 4-14: LABELING

Label the following image from the list of terms provided in the Chapter 4 Word List in Appendix B.

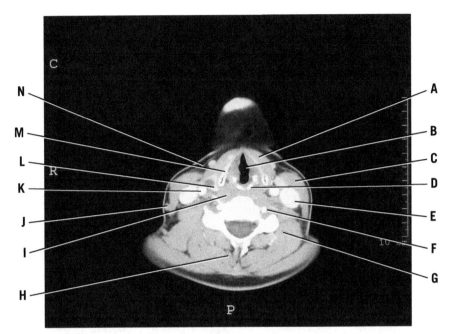

CT Images provided courtesy of Roger Williams Medical Center.

A. _____

B. _____

C. _____

D. _____

E. _____

F. _____

G. _____

H. _____

I. _____

J. _____

K. _____

L. _____

M. _____

N. _____

EXERCISE 4-15: LABELING

Label the following image from the list of terms provided in the Chapter 4 Word List in Appendix B.

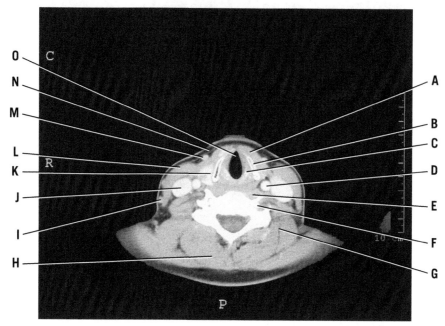

CT Images provided courtesy of Roger Williams Medical Center.

A. _____   I. _____

B. _____   J. _____

C. _____   K. _____

D. _____   L. _____

E. _____   M. _____

F. _____   N. _____

G. _____   O. _____

H. _____

EXERCISE 4-16: LABELING

Label the following image from the list of terms provided in the Chapter 4 Word List in Appendix B.

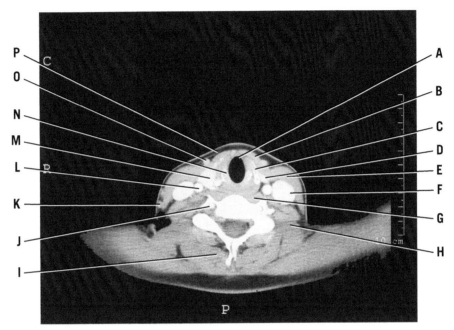

CT Images provided courtesy of Roger Williams Medical Center.

A. _____

B. _____

C. _____

D. _____

E. _____

F. _____

G. _____

H. _____

I. _____

J. _____

K. _____

L. _____

M. _____

N. _____

O. _____

P. _____

EXERCISE 4-17: LABELING

Label the following image from the list of terms provided in the Chapter 4 Word List in Appendix B.

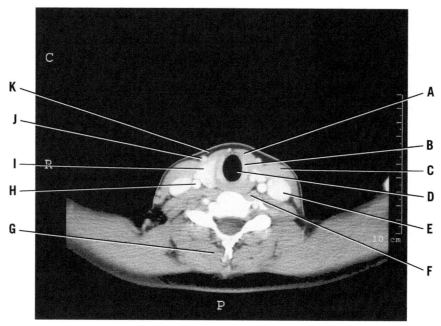

CT Images provided courtesy of Roger Williams Medical Center.

A. _____

B. _____

C. _____

D. _____

E. _____

F. _____

G. _____

H. _____

I. _____

J. _____

K. _____

EXERCISE 4-18: LABELING

Label the following image from the list of terms provided in the Chapter 4 Word List in Appendix B.

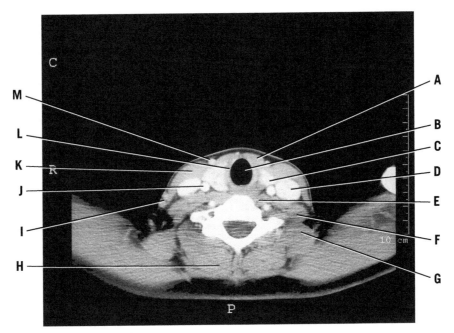

CT Images provided courtesy of Roger Williams Medical Center.

A. _____

B. _____

C. _____

D. _____

E. _____

F. _____

G. _____

H. _____

I. _____

J. _____

K. _____

L. _____

M. _____

EXERCISE 4-19: LABELING

Label the following image from the list of terms provided in the Chapter 4 Word List in Appendix B.

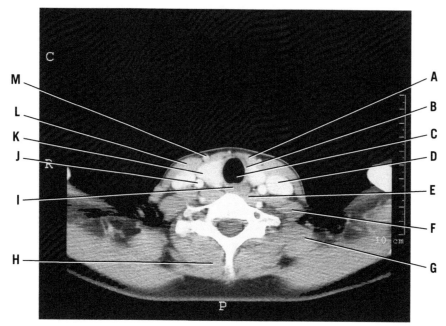

CT Images provided courtesy of Roger Williams Medical Center.

A. _____

B. _____

C. _____

D. _____

E. _____

F. _____

G. _____

H. _____

I. _____

J. _____

K. _____

L. _____

M. _____

MR IMAGES

AXIAL IMAGES

EXERCISE 4-20: LABELING

Label the following image from the list of terms provided in the Chapter 4 Word List in Appendix B.

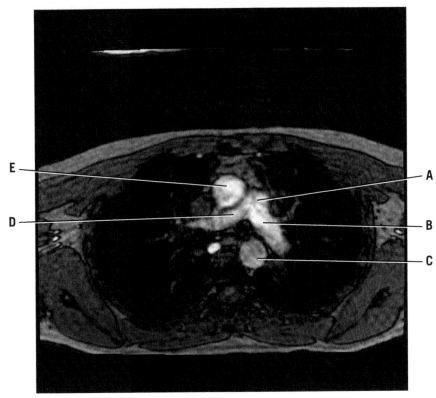

MR Images provided courtesy of Memorial Hospital of Rhode Island.

A. _____

B. _____

C. _____

D. _____

E. _____

EXERCISE 4-21: LABELING

Label the following image from the list of terms provided in the Chapter 4 Word List in Appendix B.

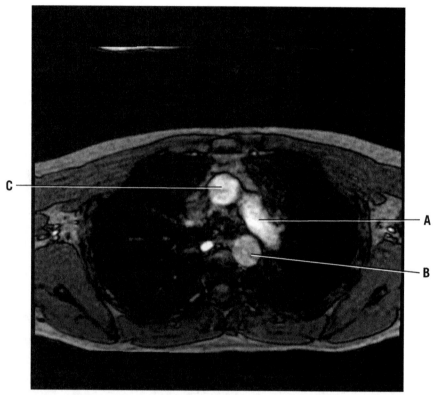

MR Images provided courtesy of Memorial Hospital of Rhode Island.

A. _____

B. _____

C. _____

EXERCISE 4-22: LABELING

Label the following image from the list of terms provided in the Chapter 4 Word List in Appendix B.

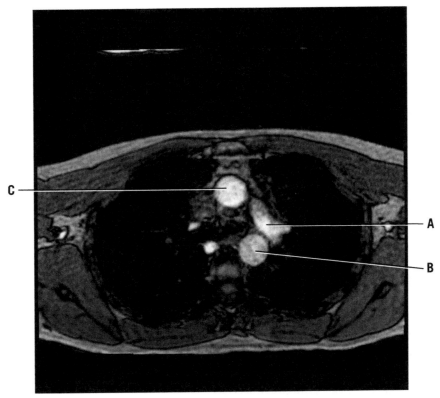

MR Images provided courtesy of Memorial Hospital of Rhode Island.

A. _____

B. _____

C. _____

EXERCISE 4-23: LABELING

Label the following image from the list of terms provided in the Chapter 4 Word List in Appendix B.

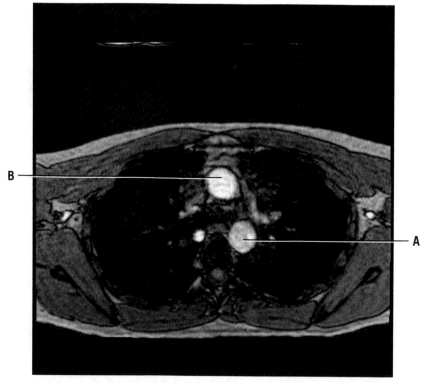

MR Images provided courtesy of Memorial Hospital of Rhode Island.

A. _____

B. _____

EXERCISE 4-24: LABELING

Label the following image from the list of terms provided in the Chapter 4 Word List in Appendix B.

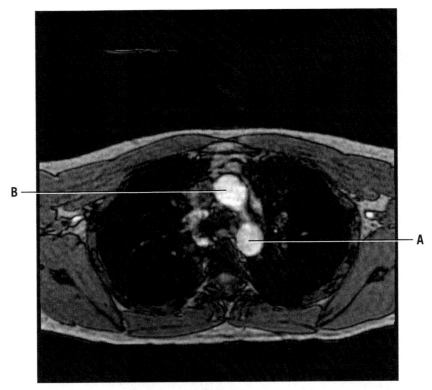

MR Images provided courtesy of Memorial Hospital of Rhode Island.

A. _____

B. _____

EXERCISE 4-25: LABELING

Label the following image from the list of terms provided in the Chapter 4 Word List in Appendix B.

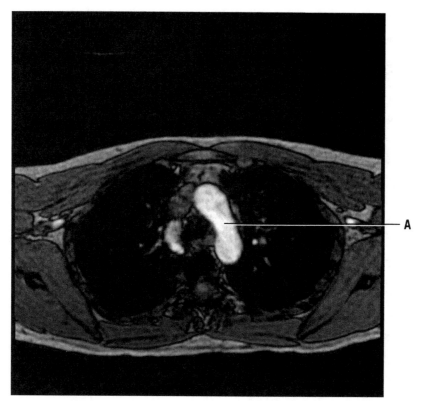

MR Images provided courtesy of Memorial Hospital of Rhode Island.

A. _____

EXERCISE 4-26: LABELING

Label the following image from the list of terms provided in the Chapter 4 Word List in Appendix B.

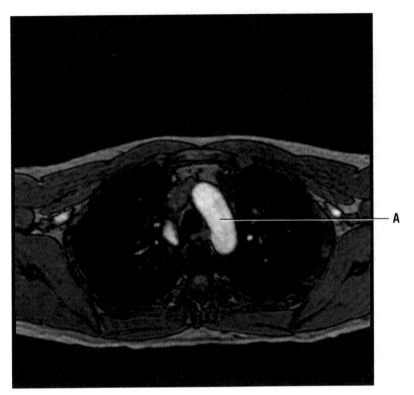

MR Images provided courtesy of Memorial Hospital of Rhode Island.

A. _____

EXERCISE 4-27: LABELING

Label the following image from the list of terms provided in the Chapter 4 Word List in Appendix B.

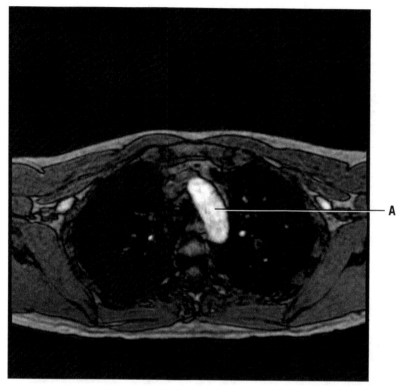

MR Images provided courtesy of Memorial Hospital of Rhode Island.

A. _____

EXERCISE 4-28: LABELING

Label the following image from the list of terms provided in the Chapter 4 Word List in Appendix B.

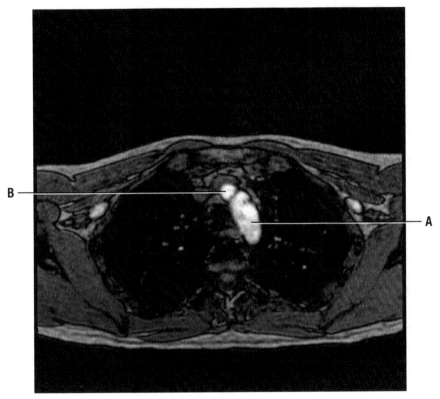

MR Images provided courtesy of Memorial Hospital of Rhode Island.

A. _____

B. _____

EXERCISE 4-29: LABELING

Label the following image from the list of terms provided in the Chapter 4 Word List in Appendix B.

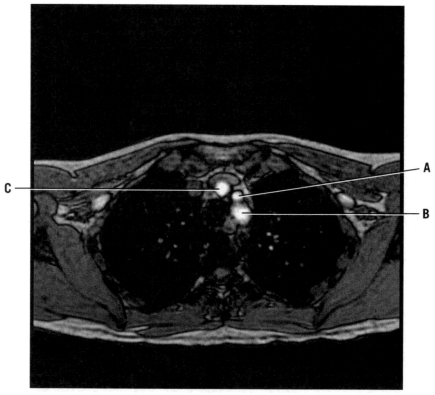

MR Images provided courtesy of Memorial Hospital of Rhode Island.

A. _____

B. _____

C. _____

EXERCISE 4-30: LABELING

Label the following image from the list of terms provided in the Chapter 4 Word List in Appendix B.

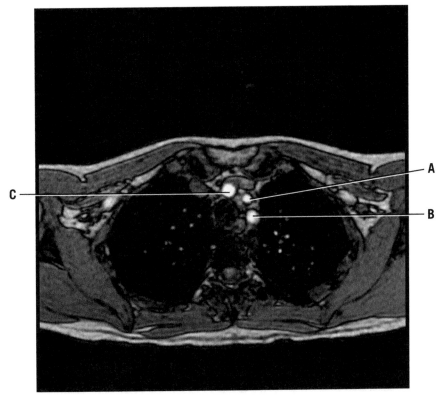

MR Images provided courtesy of Memorial Hospital of Rhode Island.

A. _____

B. _____

C. _____

EXERCISE 4-31: LABELING

Label the following image from the list of terms provided in the Chapter 4 Word List in Appendix B.

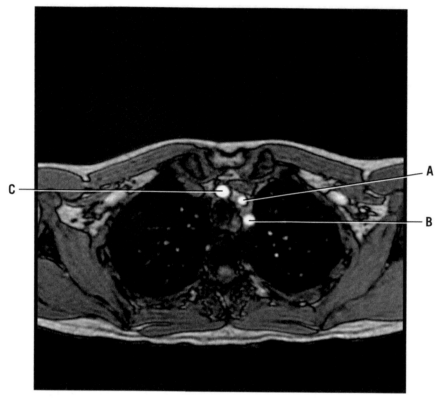

MR Images provided courtesy of Memorial Hospital of Rhode Island.

A. _____

B. _____

C. _____

EXERCISE 4-32: LABELING

Label the following image from the list of terms provided in the Chapter 4 Word List in Appendix B.

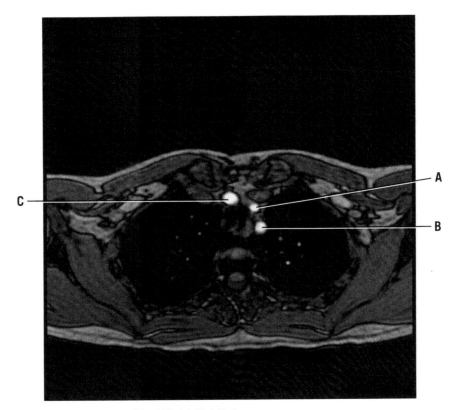

MR Images provided courtesy of Memorial Hospital of Rhode Island.

A. _____

B. _____

C. _____

EXERCISE 4-33: LABELING

Label the following image from the list of terms provided in the Chapter 4 Word List in Appendix B.

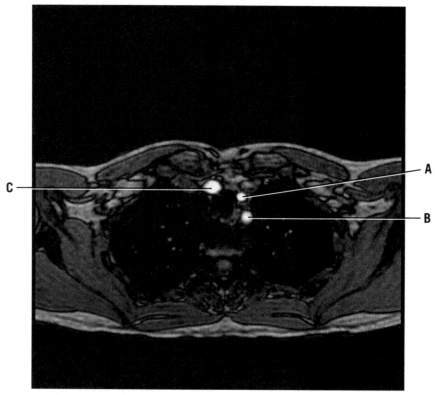

MR Images provided courtesy of Memorial Hospital of Rhode Island.

A. _____

B. _____

C. _____

EXERCISE 4-34: LABELING

Label the following image from the list of terms provided in the Chapter 4 Word List in Appendix B.

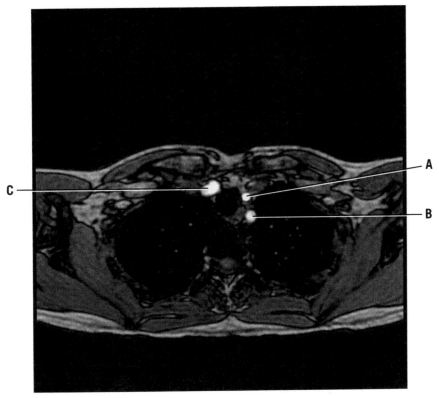

MR Images provided courtesy of Memorial Hospital of Rhode Island.

A. _____

B. _____

C. _____

EXERCISE 4-35: LABELING

Label the following image from the list of terms provided in the Chapter 4 Word List in Appendix B.

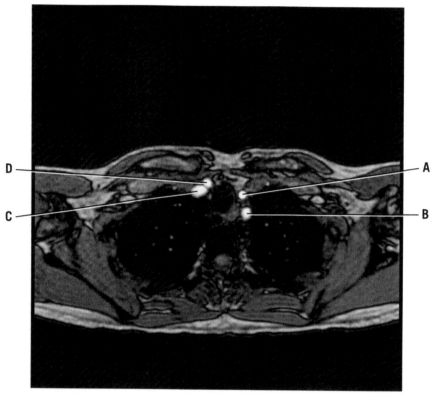

MR Images provided courtesy of Memorial Hospital of Rhode Island.

A. _____

B. _____

C. _____

D. _____

EXERCISE 4-36: LABELING

Label the following image from the list of terms provided in the Chapter 4 Word List in Appendix B.

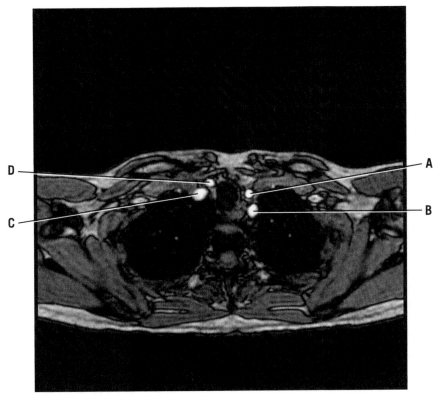

MR Images provided courtesy of Memorial Hospital of Rhode Island.

A. _____

B. _____

C. _____

D. _____

EXERCISE 4-37: LABELING

Label the following image from the list of terms provided in the Chapter 4 Word List in Appendix B.

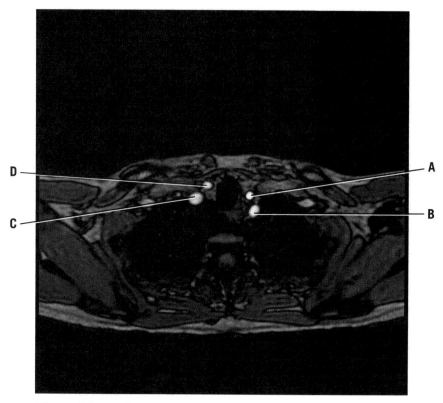

MR Images provided courtesy of Memorial Hospital of Rhode Island.

A. _____

B. _____

C. _____

D. _____

EXERCISE 4-38: LABELING

Label the following image from the list of terms provided in the Chapter 4 Word List in Appendix B.

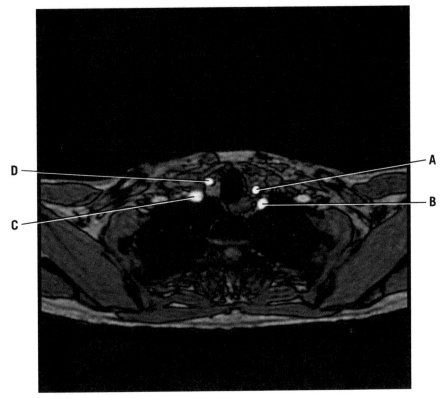

MR Images provided courtesy of Memorial Hospital of Rhode Island.

A. _____

B. _____

C. _____

D. _____

EXERCISE 4-39: LABELING

Label the following image from the list of terms provided in the Chapter 4 Word List in Appendix B.

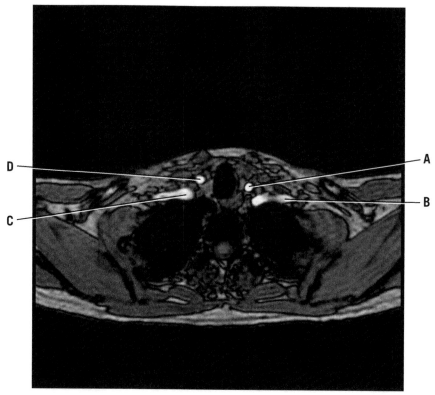

MR Images provided courtesy of Memorial Hospital of Rhode Island.

A. _____

B. _____

C. _____

D. _____

EXERCISE 4-40: LABELING

Label the following image from the list of terms provided in the Chapter 4 Word List in Appendix B.

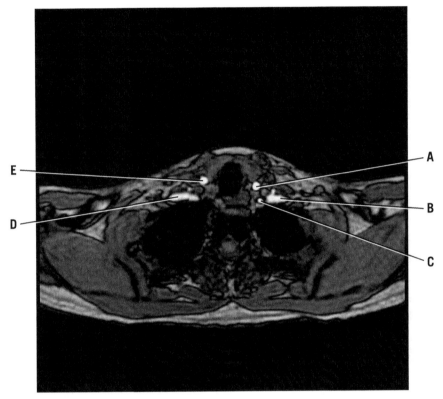

MR Images provided courtesy of Memorial Hospital of Rhode Island.

A. _____

B. _____

C. _____

D. _____

E. _____

EXERCISE 4-41: LABELING

Label the following image from the list of terms provided in the Chapter 4 Word List in Appendix B.

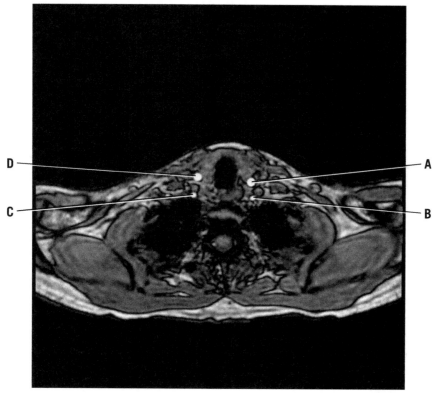

MR Images provided courtesy of Memorial Hospital of Rhode Island.

A. _____

B. _____

C. _____

D. _____

EXERCISE 4-42: LABELING

Label the following image from the list of terms provided in the Chapter 4 Word List in Appendix B.

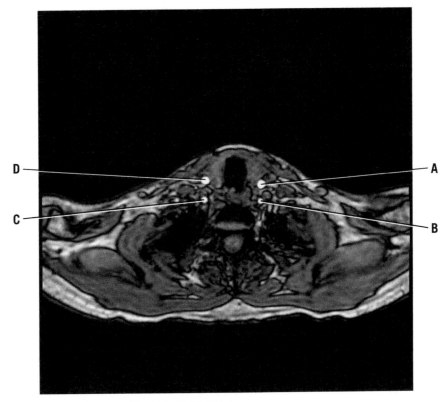

MR Images provided courtesy of Memorial Hospital of Rhode Island.

A. _____

B. _____

C. _____

D. _____

EXERCISE 4-43: LABELING

Label the following image from the list of terms provided in the Chapter 4 Word List in Appendix B.

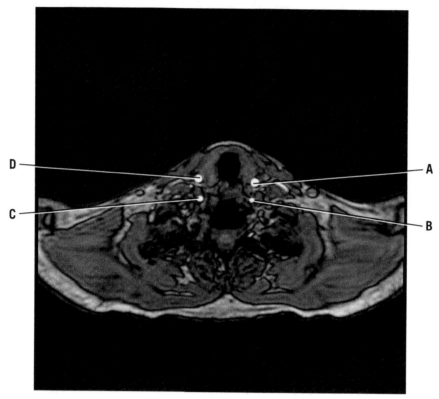

MR Images provided courtesy of Memorial Hospital of Rhode Island.

A. _____

B. _____

C. _____

D. _____

EXERCISE 4-44: LABELING

Label the following image from the list of terms provided in the Chapter 4 Word List in Appendix B.

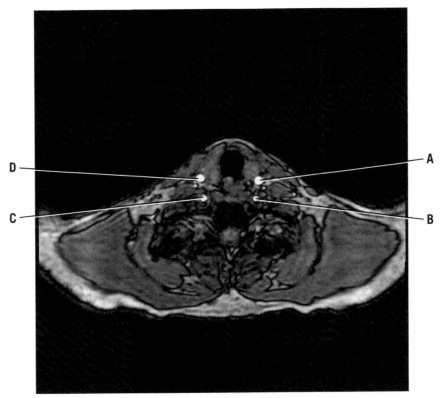

MR Images provided courtesy of Memorial Hospital of Rhode Island.

A. _____

B. _____

C. _____

D. _____

EXERCISE 4-45: LABELING

Label the following image from the list of terms provided in the Chapter 4 Word List in Appendix B.

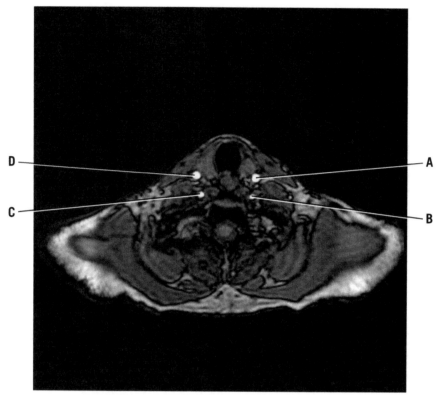

MR Images provided courtesy of Memorial Hospital of Rhode Island.

A. _____

B. _____

C. _____

D. _____

EXERCISE 4-46: LABELING

Label the following image from the list of terms provided in the Chapter 4 Word List in Appendix B.

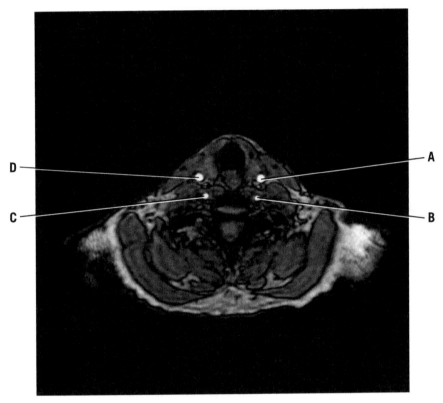

MR Images provided courtesy of Memorial Hospital of Rhode Island.

A. _____

B. _____

C. _____

D. _____

EXERCISE 4-47: LABELING

Label the following image from the list of terms provided in the Chapter 4 Word List in Appendix B.

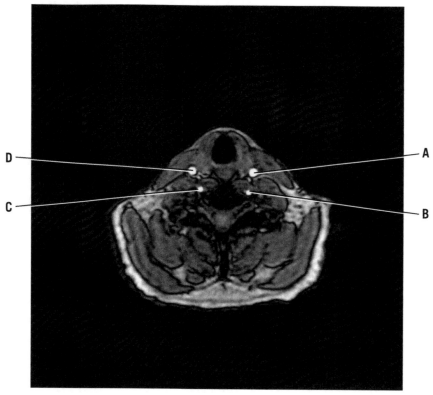

MR Images provided courtesy of Memorial Hospital of Rhode Island.

A. _____

B. _____

C. _____

D. _____

EXERCISE 4-48: LABELING

Label the following image from the list of terms provided in the Chapter 4 Word List in Appendix B.

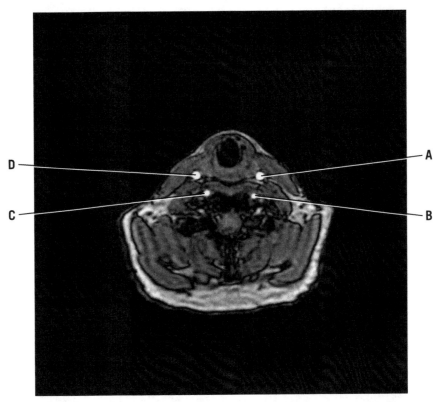

MR Images provided courtesy of Memorial Hospital of Rhode Island.

A. _____

B. _____

C. _____

D. _____

LATERAL IMAGE

EXERCISE 4-49: LABELING

Label the following image from the list of terms provided in the Chapter 4 Word List in Appendix B.

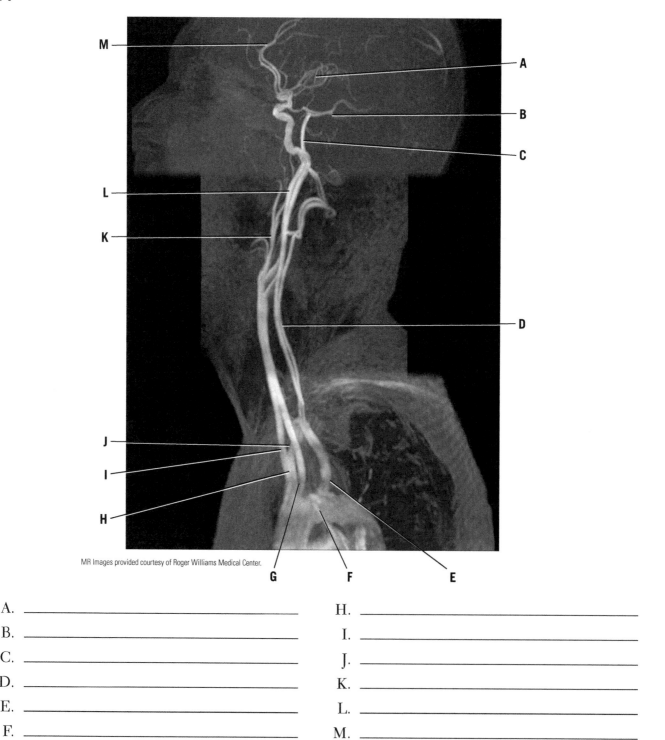

MR Images provided courtesy of Roger Williams Medical Center.

A. _____   H. _____

B. _____   I. _____

C. _____   J. _____

D. _____   K. _____

E. _____   L. _____

F. _____   M. _____

G. _____

CORONAL IMAGE

EXERCISE 4-50: LABELING

Label the following image from the list of terms provided in the Chapter 4 Word List in Appendix B.

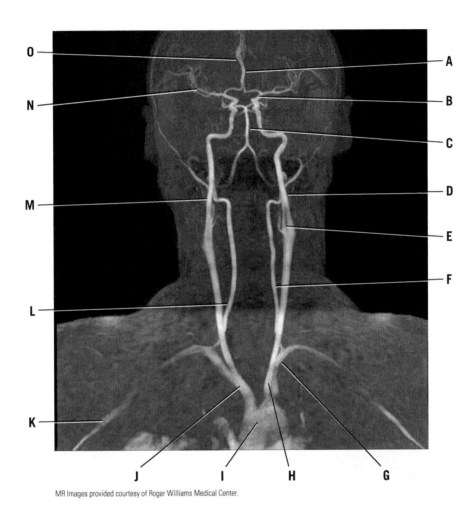

MR Images provided courtesy of Roger Williams Medical Center.

A. _____   I. _____

B. _____   J. _____

C. _____   K. _____

D. _____   L. _____

E. _____   M. _____

F. _____   N. _____

G. _____   O. _____

H. _____

CIRCLE OF WILLIS

EXERCISE 4-51: LABELING

Label the following image from the list of terms provided in the Chapter 4 Word List in Appendix B.

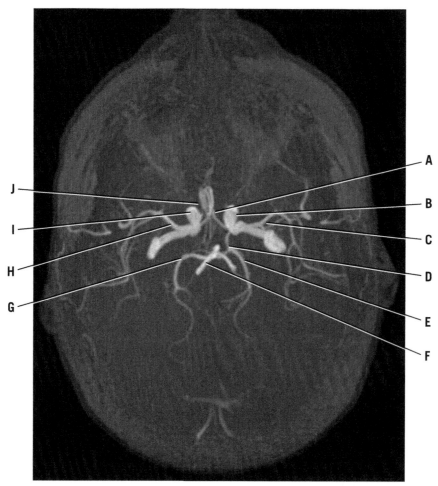

MR Images provided courtesy of Roger Williams Medical Center.

A. _____   F. _____

B. _____   G. _____

C. _____   H. _____

D. _____   I. _____

E. _____   J. _____

Thorax

OUTLINE

EXERCISE 5-1: LABELING

Label the following illustration from the list of terms provided.

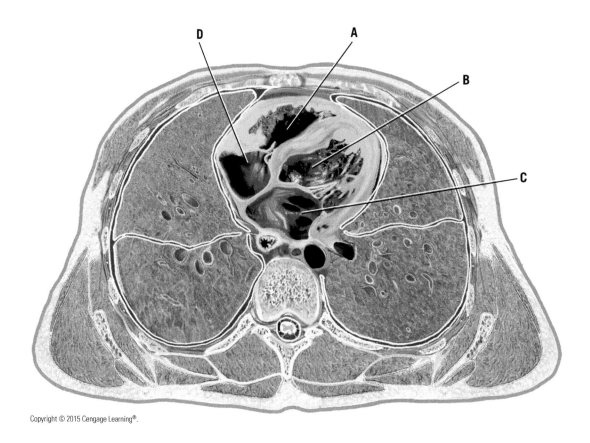

left atrium
left ventricle
right atrium
right ventricle

A. _____

B. _____

C. _____

D. _____

EXERCISE 5-2: MATCHING

Match the following terms with the correct definitions.

____ 1. mitral valve

____ 2. semilunar valve

____ 3. thebesian valve

____ 4. tricuspid valve

a. a valve having three cusps or flaps found on the right side of the heart between the right atrium and right ventricle

b. a valve having two cusps or flaps found on the left side of the heart between the left atrium and left ventricle

c. crescent or half-moon-shaped valve

d. the valve controlling blood flow from the coronary sinus into the right atrium of the heart

EXERCISE 5-3: TERM IDENTIFICATION

Provide the correct term for the following definitions.

1. a large indentation along the medial left lung accommodating the heart   _____

2. the inferior segment of the sternum   _____

3. an opening between the right and left atria of the heart in the fetus   _____

4. the palpable joint between the manubrium and body or gladiolus of the sternum   _____

5. referring to a viscus or an organ within a cavity   _____

EXERCISE 5-4: IDENTIFICATION

Identify the great vessels.

1. _____
2. _____
3. _____
4. _____

EXERCISE 5-5: TERM IDENTIFICATION

Provide an alternate term for the following terms.

1. jugular notch   _____

2. mitral valve   _____

3. visceral layer of the serous pericardium   _____

4. xiphoid process   _____

EXERCISE 5-6: LABELING

Label the following illustration from the list of terms provided.

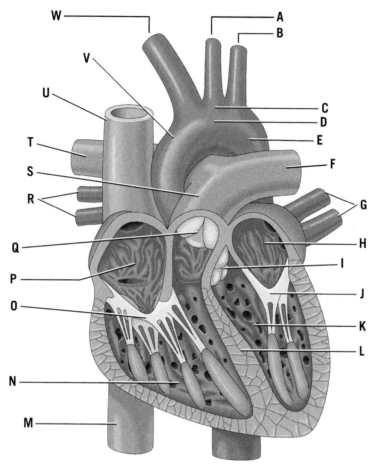

Copyright © 2015 Cengage Learning®.

aorta
aortic arch
aortic semilunar valve
ascending aorta
bicuspid (mitral) valve
brachiocephalic artery
descending aorta
inferior vena cava
left atrium
left common carotid artery
left pulmonary artery
left pulmonary veins
left subclavian artery
left ventricle
pulmonary semilunar valve
pulmonary trunk
right atrium
right pulmonary artery
right pulmonary veins
right ventricle
septum
superior vena cava
tricuspid valve

A. _____

B. _____

C. _____

D. _____

E. _____

F. _____

G. _____

H. _____

I. _____

J. _____

K. _____

L. _____

M. _____

N. _____

O. _____

P. _____

Q. _____

R. _____

S. _____

T. _____

U. _____

V. _____

W. _____

EXERCISE 5-7: ABBREVIATIONS

Provide the meaning for the following abbreviations.

1. IVC _____

2. SC _____

3. SVC _____

EXERCISE 5-8: LABELING

Label the following illustration from the list of terms provided.

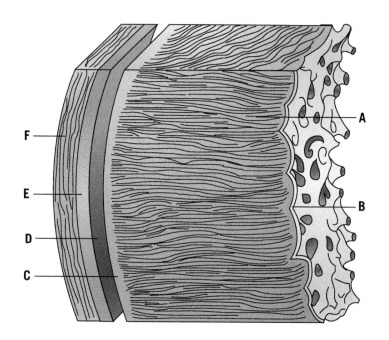

endocardium
fibrous pericardium
myocardium
serous pericardium (parietal layer)
serous pericardium (visceral layer)
   (epicardium)
space

A. _____

B. _____

C. _____

D. _____

E. _____

F. _____

EXERCISE 5-9: COMPLETION

Fill in the following blanks by selecting the correct terms from the list provided. (Some terms may be used more than once.)

alveoli
aorta
aortic semilunar valve
bicuspid valve
capillaries
coronary sinus
deoxygenated
IVC

left atrium
left ventricle
lungs
mitral valve
oxygenated
pulmonary arteries
pulmonary circulatory system
pulmonary semilunar valve

pulmonary trunk
pulmonary veins
right atrium
right ventricle
SVC
systemic circulatory system
tricuspid valve

Blood Flow of the Heart

Three vessels, carrying _____ blood, drain into the

_____ of the heart. They are the _____,

_____, and _____ . From there, the blood

passes through the _____ into the _____ and then

out of the heart via the _____, first passing through the

_____. This is the start of the _____. The

_____ bifurcates into the _____, heading toward

the _____. Once there, the vessels break down into the smallest vessels,

the _____, surrounding the _____, where diffusion

occurs. The vessels eventually become the _____, leave the lungs, and

enter the _____ of the heart, carrying _____

blood. From there, the blood passes through the _____, or

_____, into the _____, and then exits via the

_____, passing first through the _____ . This is the

beginning of the _____.

EXERCISE 5-10: SORTING

Arrange the following in the order that they occur, looking at sectional images in descending order.

A. The right atrium and left atrium appear.

B. The pulmonary trunk is seen with its two branches, the right and left pulmonary arteries, as well as the split of the trachea into the right and left bronchi.

C. The left brachiocephalic vein passes transversely to join with the right.

D. The brachiocephalic veins are seen on either side of the right brachiocephalic artery, left common carotid artery, and left subclavian artery.

E. The IVC appears.

1. ___

2. ___

3. ___

4. ___

5. ___

EXERCISE 5-11: IDENTIFICATION

Categorize each of the following muscles as belonging to the (A) anterior thoracic region, (B) lateral thoracic region, (C) posterior thoracic region, or (D) muscles of the thorax.

___ 1. trapezius

___ 2. levator scapulae

___ 3. serratus anterior

___ 4. pectoralis (major and minor)

___ 5. intercostal (external and internal)

___ 6. rhomboid (major and minor)

___ 7. splenius capitis and colli

___ 8. diaphragm

___ 9. subclavius

___ 10. serratus posterior (superior and inferior)

CT AXIAL IMAGES

EXERCISE 5-12: LABELING

Label the following image from the list of terms provided in the **Chapter 5 Word List in Appendix B.**

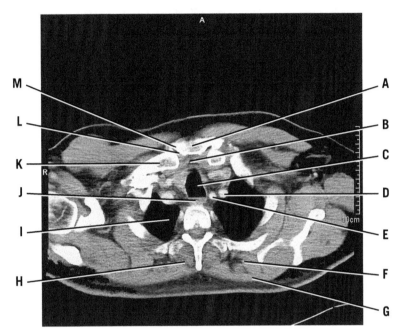

CT images provided by Our Lady of Fatima Hospital, North Providence, Rhode Island.

A. _____

B. _____

C. _____

D. _____

E. _____

F. _____

G. _____

H. _____

I. _____

J. _____

K. _____

L. _____

M. _____

EXERCISE 5-13: LABELING

Label the following image from the list of terms provided in the Chapter 5 Word List in Appendix B.

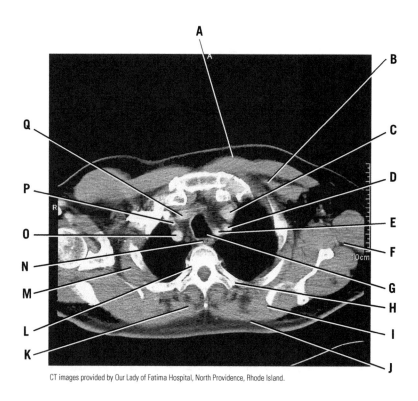

CT images provided by Our Lady of Fatima Hospital, North Providence, Rhode Island.

A. _____   J. _____

B. _____   K. _____

C. _____   L. _____

D. _____   M. _____

E. _____   N. _____

F. _____   O. _____

G. _____   P. _____

H. _____   Q. _____

I. _____

EXERCISE 5-14: LABELING

Label the following image from the list of terms provided in the Chapter 5 Word List in Appendix B.

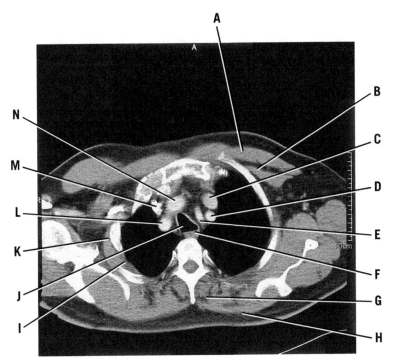

CT images provided by Our Lady of Fatima Hospital, North Providence, Rhode Island.

A. _____

B. _____

C. _____

D. _____

E. _____

F. _____

G. _____

H. _____

I. _____

J. _____

K. _____

L. _____

M. _____

N. _____

EXERCISE 5-15: LABELING

Label the following image from the list of terms provided in the Chapter 5 Word List in Appendix B.

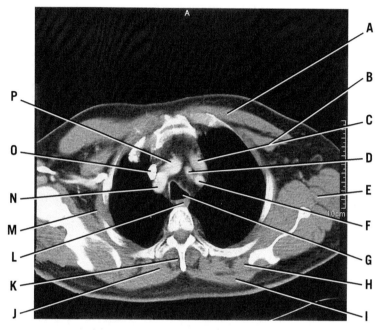

CT images provided by Our Lady of Fatima Hospital, North Providence, Rhode Island.

A. _____

B. _____

C. _____

D. _____

E. _____

F. _____

G. _____

H. _____

I. _____

J. _____

K. _____

L. _____

M. _____

N. _____

O. _____

P. _____

EXERCISE 5-16: LABELING

Label the following image from the list of terms provided in the Chapter 5 Word List in Appendix B.

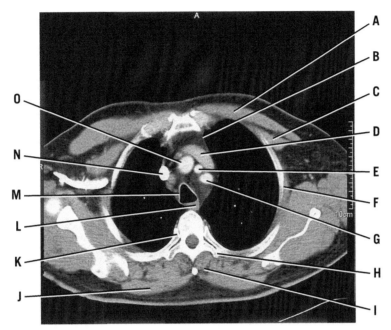

CT images provided by Our Lady of Fatima Hospital, North Providence, Rhode Island.

A. _____

B. _____

C. _____

D. _____

E. _____

F. _____

G. _____

H. _____

I. _____

J. _____

K. _____

L. _____

M. _____

N. _____

O. _____

EXERCISE 5-17: LABELING

Label the following image from the list of terms provided in the Chapter 5 Word List in Appendix B.

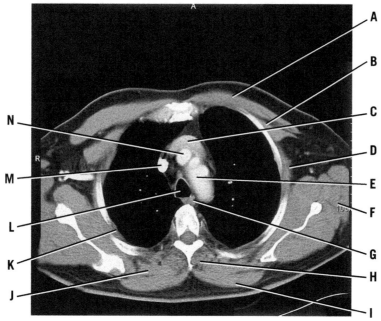

CT images provided by Our Lady of Fatima Hospital, North Providence, Rhode Island.

A. _____   H. _____

B. _____   I. _____

C. _____   J. _____

D. _____   K. _____

E. _____   L. _____

F. _____   M. _____

G. _____   N. _____

EXERCISE 5-18: LABELING

Label the following image from the list of terms provided in the Chapter 5 Word List in Appendix B.

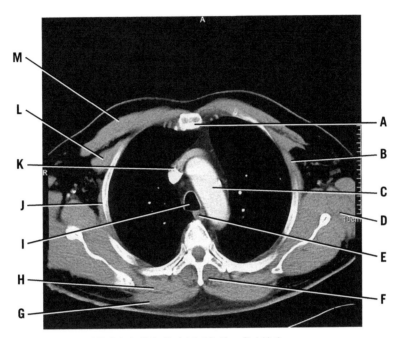

CT images provided by Our Lady of Fatima Hospital, North Providence, Rhode Island.

A. _____

B. _____

C. _____

D. _____

E. _____

F. _____

G. _____

H. _____

I. _____

J. _____

K. _____

L. _____

M. _____

EXERCISE 5-19: LABELING

Label the following image from the list of terms provided in the Chapter 5 Word List in Appendix B.

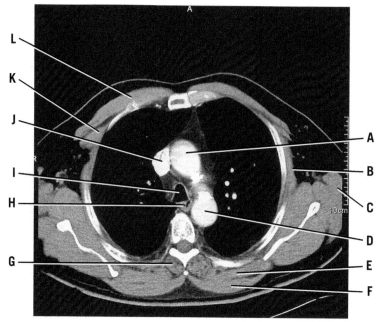

CT images provided by Our Lady of Fatima Hospital, North Providence, Rhode Island.

A. _____

B. _____

C. _____

D. _____

E. _____

F. _____

G. _____

H. _____

I. _____

J. _____

K. _____

L. _____

EXERCISE 5-20: LABELING

Label the following image from the list of terms provided in the Chapter 5 Word List in Appendix B.

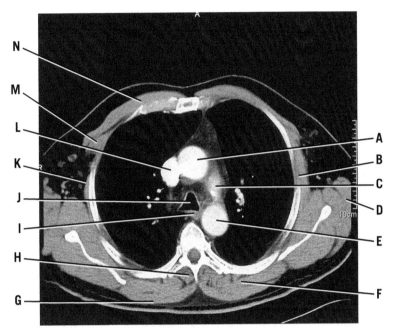

CT images provided by Our Lady of Fatima Hospital, North Providence, Rhode Island.

A. _____

B. _____

C. _____

D. _____

E. _____

F. _____

G. _____

H. _____

I. _____

J. _____

K. _____

L. _____

M. _____

N. _____

EXERCISE 5-21: LABELING

Label the following image from the list of terms provided in the Chapter 5 Word List in Appendix B.

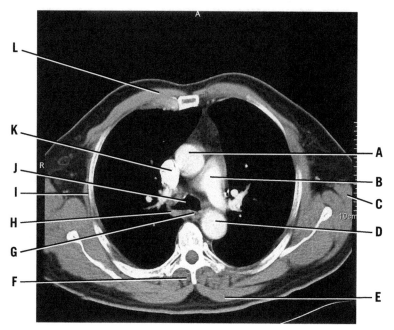

CT images provided by Our Lady of Fatima Hospital, North Providence, Rhode Island.

A. _____

B. _____

C. _____

D. _____

E. _____

F. _____

G. _____

H. _____

I. _____

J. _____

K. _____

L. _____

EXERCISE 5-22: LABELING

Label the following image from the list of terms provided in the Chapter 5 Word List in Appendix B.

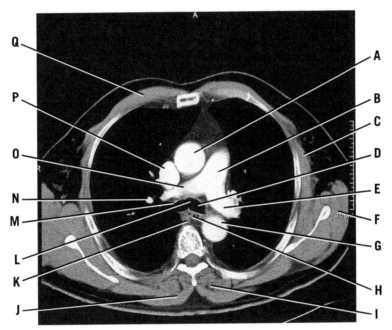

CT images provided by Our Lady of Fatima Hospital, North Providence, Rhode Island.

A. _____

B. _____

C. _____

D. _____

E. _____

F. _____

G. _____

H. _____

I. _____

J. _____

K. _____

L. _____

M. _____

N. _____

O. _____

P. _____

Q. _____

EXERCISE 5-23: LABELING

Label the following image from the list of terms provided in the Chapter 5 Word List in Appendix B.

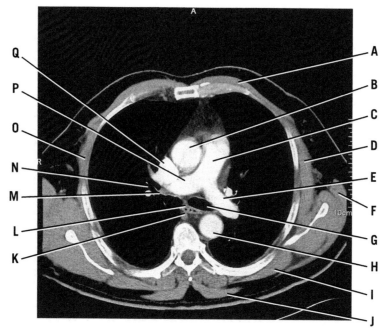

CT images provided by Our Lady of Fatima Hospital, North Providence, Rhode Island.

A. _____

B. _____

C. _____

D. _____

E. _____

F. _____

G. _____

H. _____

I. _____

J. _____

K. _____

L. _____

M. _____

N. _____

O. _____

P. _____

Q. _____

EXERCISE 5-24: LABELING

Label the following image from the list of terms provided in the Chapter 5 Word List in Appendix B.

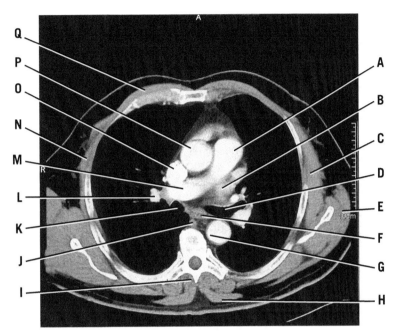

CT images provided by Our Lady of Fatima Hospital, North Providence, Rhode Island.

A. _____

B. _____

C. _____

D. _____

E. _____

F. _____

G. _____

H. _____

I. _____

J. _____

K. _____

L. _____

M. _____

N. _____

O. _____

P. _____

Q. _____

EXERCISE 5-25: LABELING

Label the following image from the list of terms provided in the Chapter 5 Word List in Appendix B.

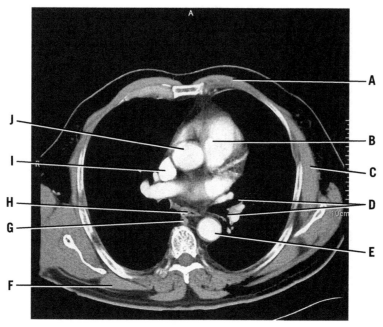

CT images provided by Our Lady of Fatima Hospital, North Providence, Rhode Island.

A. _____

B. _____

C. _____

D. _____

E. _____

F. _____

G. _____

H. _____

I. _____

J. _____

EXERCISE 5-26: LABELING

Label the following image from the list of terms provided in the Chapter 5 Word List in Appendix B.

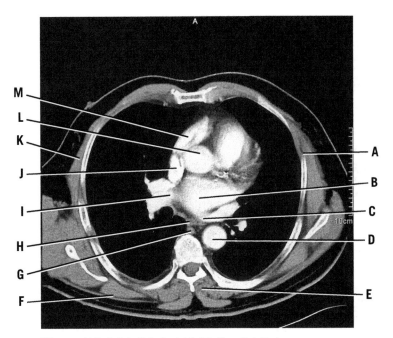

CT images provided by Our Lady of Fatima Hospital, North Providence, Rhode Island.

A. _____

B. _____

C. _____

D. _____

E. _____

F. _____

G. _____

H. _____

I. _____

J. _____

K. _____

L. _____

M. _____

EXERCISE 5-27: LABELING

Label the following image from the list of terms provided in the Chapter 5 Word List in Appendix B.

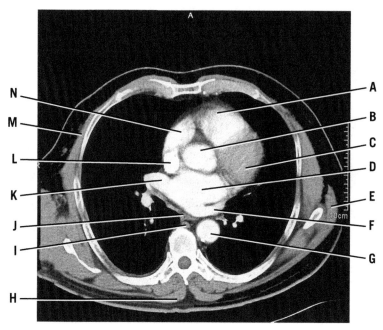

CT images provided by Our Lady of Fatima Hospital, North Providence, Rhode Island.

A. _____

B. _____

C. _____

D. _____

E. _____

F. _____

G. _____

H. _____

I. _____

J. _____

K. _____

L. _____

M. _____

N. _____

EXERCISE 5-28: LABELING

Label the following image from the list of terms provided in the Chapter 5 Word List in Appendix B.

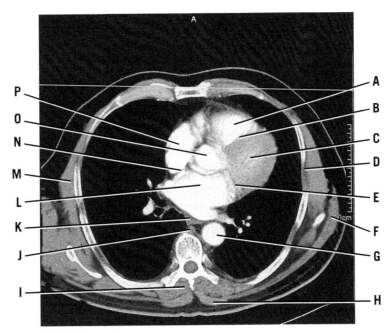

CT images provided by Our Lady of Fatima Hospital, North Providence, Rhode Island.

A. _____   I. _____

B. _____   J. _____

C. _____   K. _____

D. _____   L. _____

E. _____   M. _____

F. _____   N. _____

G. _____   O. _____

H. _____   P. _____

EXERCISE 5-29: LABELING

Label the following image from the list of terms provided in the Chapter 5 Word List in Appendix B.

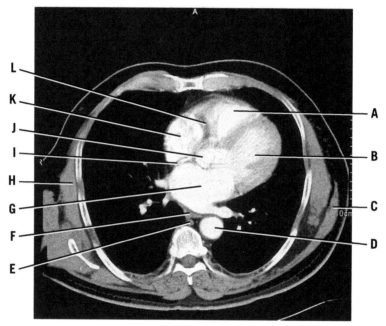

CT images provided by Our Lady of Fatima Hospital, North Providence, Rhode Island.

A. _____

B. _____

C. _____

D. _____

E. _____

F. _____

G. _____

H. _____

I. _____

J. _____

K. _____

L. _____

EXERCISE 5-30: LABELING

Label the following image from the list of terms provided in the Chapter 5 Word List in Appendix B.

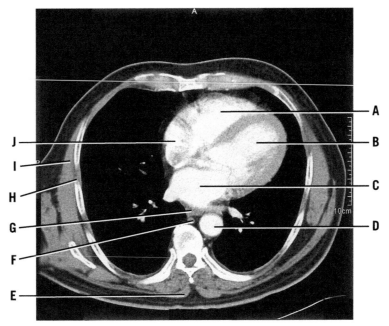

CT images provided by Our Lady of Fatima Hospital, North Providence, Rhode Island.

A. _____

B. _____

C. _____

D. _____

E. _____

F. _____

G. _____

H. _____

I. _____

J. _____

EXERCISE 5-31: LABELING

Label the following image from the list of terms provided in the Chapter 5 Word List in Appendix B.

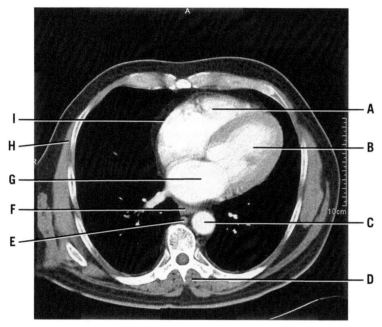

CT images provided by Our Lady of Fatima Hospital, North Providence, Rhode Island.

A. _____

B. _____

C. _____

D. _____

E. _____

F. _____

G. _____

H. _____

I. _____

EXERCISE 5-32: LABELING

Label the following image from the list of terms provided in the Chapter 5 Word List in Appendix B.

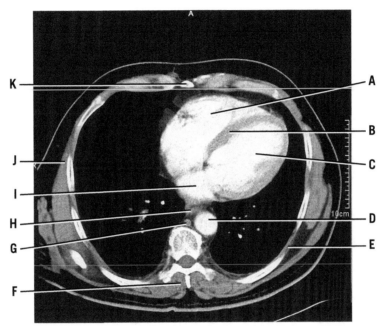

CT images provided by Our Lady of Fatima Hospital, North Providence, Rhode Island.

A. _____

B. _____

C. _____

D. _____

E. _____

F. _____

G. _____

H. _____

I. _____

J. _____

K. _____

EXERCISE 5-33: LABELING

Label the following image from the list of terms provided in the Chapter 5 Word List in Appendix B.

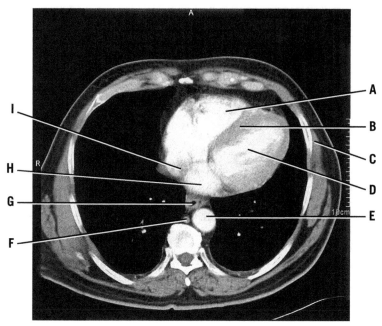

CT images provided by Our Lady of Fatima Hospital, North Providence, Rhode Island.

A. _____

B. _____

C. _____

D. _____

E. _____

F. _____

G. _____

H. _____

I. _____

EXERCISE 5-34: LABELING

Label the following image from the list of terms provided in the Chapter 5 Word List in Appendix B.

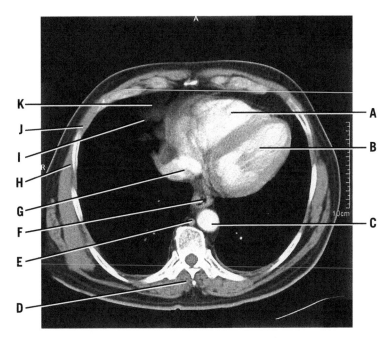

CT images provided by Our Lady of Fatima Hospital, North Providence, Rhode Island.

A. _____

B. _____

C. _____

D. _____

E. _____

F. _____

G. _____

H. _____

I. _____

J. _____

K. _____

Abdomen

OUTLINE

EXERCISE 6-1: IDENTIFICATION

Identify the three openings in the diaphragm, listing them from anterior to posterior.

1. _____
2. _____
3. _____

EXERCISE 6-2: IDENTIFICATION

Identify the major vessels arising from the abdominal descending aorta, listing them in the order they generally appear.

1. _____
2. _____
3. _____
4. _____

EXERCISE 6-3: IDENTIFICATION

Identify the three branches off of the celiac axis.

1. _____
2. _____
3. _____

EXERCISE 6-4: IDENTIFICATION

Identify the two main vessels involved in forming the portal vein.

1. _____
2. _____

EXERCISE 6-5: MATCHING

Match the following terms with the correct definition.

_____ 1. ampulla of Vater

_____ 2. cardiac notch

_____ 3. caudate lobe

_____ 4. cholelith

_____ 5. cystic duct

_____ 6. fundus

_____ 7. IMA

_____ 8. linea alba

_____ 9. pyloric antrum

_____ 10. umbilical notch

a. a large indentation along the medial left lung that accommodates the heart

b. the most inferior branch off of the abdominal descending aorta

c. a structure that drains bile from the gallbladder

d. a bulge found in the distal portion of the stomach

e. one of four lobes of the liver, found anterior to the IVC

f. the larger part of a hollow organ located farthest from the opening

g. an indentation on the anterior inferior liver

h. a tendinous membrane that separates the bilateral rectus abdominis muscles

i. a dilatation at the end of the common bile duct where it enters the duodenum

j. a gallstone

EXERCISE 6-6: IDENTIFICATION

Identify the four lobes of the liver.

1. _____

2. _____

3. _____

4. _____

EXERCISE 6-7: MATCHING

Match the following definitions with the correct term. (Some of the terms will be used more than once.)

_____ 1. attaches the liver to the anterior abdominal wall and diaphragm

_____ 2. remnant of obliterated ductus venosus

_____ 3. remnant of the umbilical vein

_____ 4. round ligament

_____ 5. separates the caudate and left lobes of the liver

_____ 6. separates the quadrate and left lobes of the liver

a. falciform ligament

b. ligamentum venosum

c. ligamentum teres

EXERCISE 6-8: LABELING

Label the following illustration from the list of terms provided.

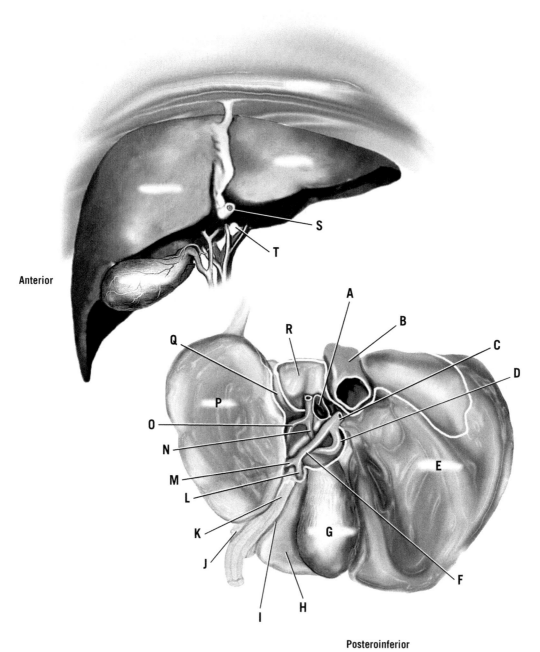

caudate lobe

common bile duct

common hepatic duct

cystic duct

falciform ligament

gallbladder

hepatic portal vein

inferior vena cava

left hepatic artery

left hepatic duct

left lobe

ligamentum teres

ligamentum venosum

longitudinal fissure

quadrate lobe

right hepatic artery

right hepatic duct

right lobe

round ligament

umbilical notch

A. _____

B. _____

C. _____

D. _____

E. _____

F. _____

G. _____

H. _____

I. _____

J. _____

K. _____

L. _____

M. _____

N. _____

O. _____

P. _____

Q. _____

R. _____

S. _____

T. _____

EXERCISE 6-9: MATCHING

Match the following sections of the small intestine with the correct location.

____ 1. duodenum

____ 2. ileum

____ 3. jejunum

a. umbilical region

b. distal portion at L4

c. hypogastric region

EXERCISE 6-10: IDENTIFICATION

Indicate whether the following are supplied by the (A) SMA or (B) IMA.

____ 1. ascending colon

____ 2. descending colon

____ 3. right half of transverse colon

____ 4. small intestine

EXERCISE 6-11: LABELING

Label the following illustration from the list of terms provided.

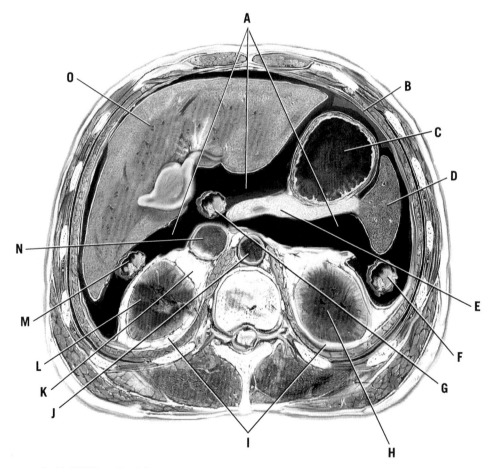

anterior pararenal compartment

aorta

ascending colon

descending colon

duodenum

inferior vena cava

left kidney

liver

pancreas

perirenal space

peritoneum

posterior pararenal compartment

right kidney

spleen

stomach

A. _____

B. _____

C. _____

D. _____

E. _____

F. _____

G. _____

H. _____

I. _____

J. _____

K. _____

L. _____

M. _____

N. _____

O. _____

EXERCISE 6-12: IDENTIFICATION

For the following, indicate whether they are in the (A) peritoneal cavity, (B) anterior pararenal space, (C) perirenal space, or (D) posterior pararenal space.

____ 1. adrenals

____ 2. aorta

____ 3. ascending colon

____ 4. descending aorta

____ 5. duodenum

____ 6. gallbladder

____ 7. kidneys

____ 8. liver

____ 9. most of the intestines

____ 10. pancreas

____ 11. spleen

____ 12. stomach

____ 13. ureters

EXERCISE 6-13: IDENTIFICATION

Indicate whether the following muscles are (A) constant in the abdominal and pelvic region or (B) unique to the abdominal region.

____ 1. erector spinae

____ 2. external oblique

____ 3. iliacus

____ 4. internal oblique

____ 5. quadratus lumborum

____ 6. rectus abdominis

____ 7. transversus abdominis

CT AXIAL IMAGES

EXERCISE 6-14: LABELING

Label the following image from the list of terms provided in the Chapter 6 Word List in Appendix B.

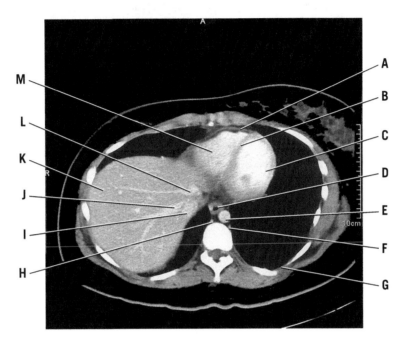

CT images provided by Our Lady of Fatima Hospital, North Providence, Rhode Island.

A. _____

B. _____

C. _____

D. _____

E. _____

F. _____

G. _____

H. _____

I. _____

J. _____

K. _____

L. _____

M. _____

EXERCISE 6-15: LABELING

Label the following image from the list of terms provided in the Chapter 6 Word List in Appendix B.

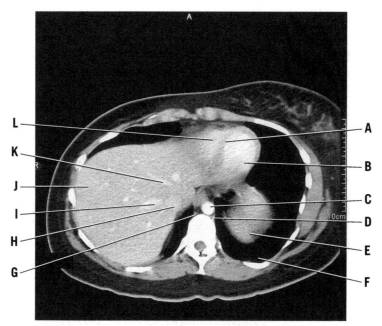

CT images provided by Our Lady of Fatima Hospital, North Providence, Rhode Island.

A. _____

B. _____

C. _____

D. _____

E. _____

F. _____

G. _____

H. _____

I. _____

J. _____

K. _____

L. _____

EXERCISE 6-16: LABELING

Label the following image from the list of terms provided in the Chapter 6 Word List in Appendix B.

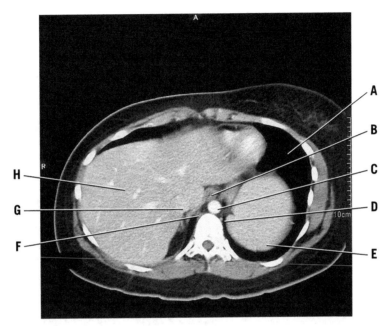

CT images provided by Our Lady of Fatima Hospital, North Providence, Rhode Island.

A. _____

B. _____

C. _____

D. _____

E. _____

F. _____

G. _____

H. _____

EXERCISE 6-17: LABELING

Label the following image from the list of terms provided in the Chapter 6 Word List in Appendix B.

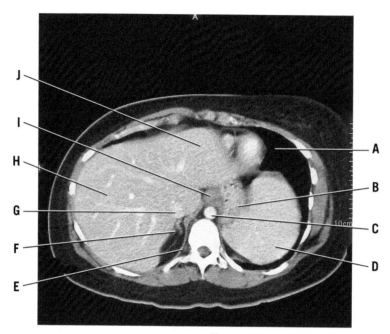

CT images provided by Our Lady of Fatima Hospital, North Providence, Rhode Island.

A. _____

B. _____

C. _____

D. _____

E. _____

F. _____

G. _____

H. _____

I. _____

J. _____

EXERCISE 6-18: LABELING

Label the following image from the list of terms provided in the Chapter 6 Word List in Appendix B.

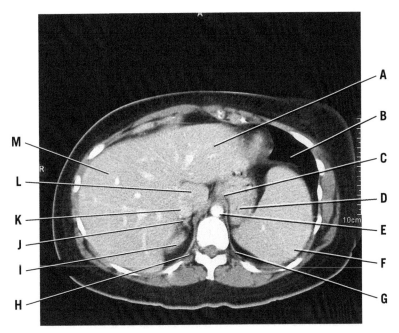

CT images provided by Our Lady of Fatima Hospital, North Providence, Rhode Island.

A. _____

B. _____

C. _____

D. _____

E. _____

F. _____

G. _____

H. _____

I. _____

J. _____

K. _____

L. _____

M. _____

EXERCISE 6-19: LABELING

Label the following image from the list of terms provided in the Chapter 6 Word List in Appendix B.

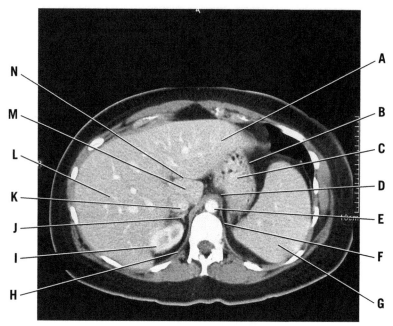

CT images provided by Our Lady of Fatima Hospital, North Providence, Rhode Island.

A. _____

B. _____

C. _____

D. _____

E. _____

F. _____

G. _____

H. _____

I. _____

J. _____

K. _____

L. _____

M. _____

N. _____

EXERCISE 6-20: LABELING

Label the following image from the list of terms provided in the Chapter 6 Word List in Appendix B.

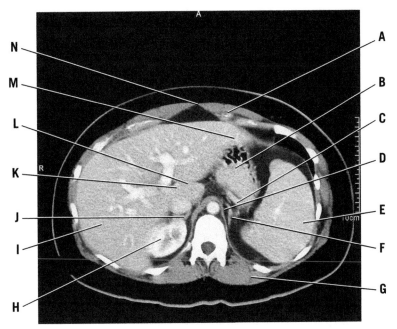

CT images provided by Our Lady of Fatima Hospital, North Providence, Rhode Island.

A. _____

B. _____

C. _____

D. _____

E. _____

F. _____

G. _____

H. _____

I. _____

J. _____

K. _____

L. _____

M. _____

N. _____

EXERCISE 6-21: LABELING

Label the following image from the list of terms provided in the Chapter 6 Word List in Appendix B.

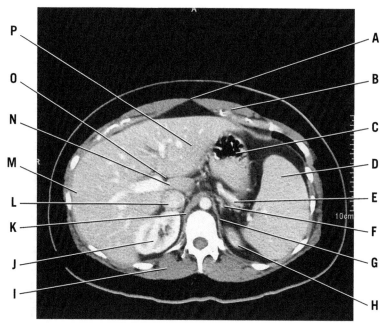

CT images provided by Our Lady of Fatima Hospital, North Providence, Rhode Island.

A. _____   I. _____

B. _____   J. _____

C. _____   K. _____

D. _____   L. _____

E. _____   M. _____

F. _____   N. _____

G. _____   O. _____

H. _____   P. _____

EXERCISE 6-22: LABELING

Label the following image from the list of terms provided in the Chapter 6 Word List in Appendix B.

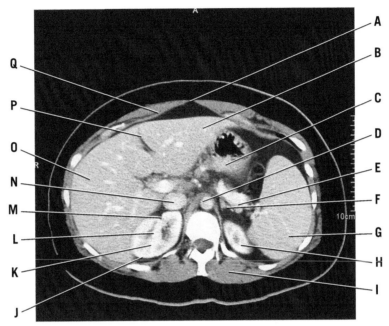

CT images provided by Our Lady of Fatima Hospital, North Providence, Rhode Island.

A. _____ J. _____

B. _____ K. _____

C. _____ L. _____

D. _____ M. _____

E. _____ N. _____

F. _____ O. _____

G. _____ P. _____

H. _____ Q. _____

I. _____

EXERCISE 6-23: LABELING

Label the following image from the list of terms provided in the Chapter 6 Word List in Appendix B.

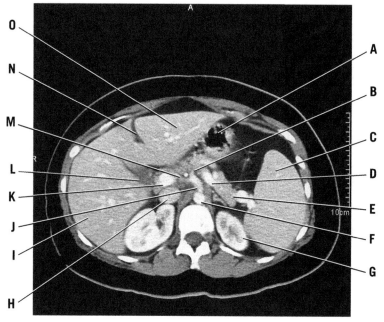

CT images provided by Our Lady of Fatima Hospital, North Providence, Rhode Island.

A. _____   I. _____

B. _____   J. _____

C. _____   K. _____

D. _____   L. _____

E. _____   M. _____

F. _____   N. _____

G. _____   O. _____

H. _____

EXERCISE 6-24: LABELING

Label the following image from the list of terms provided in the Chapter 6 Word List in Appendix B.

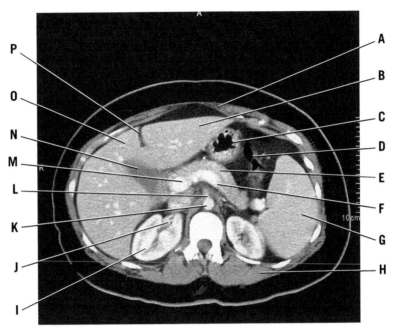

CT images provided by Our Lady of Fatima Hospital, North Providence, Rhode Island.

A. _____   I. _____

B. _____   J. _____

C. _____   K. _____

D. _____   L. _____

E. _____   M. _____

F. _____   N. _____

G. _____   O. _____

H. _____   P. _____

EXERCISE 6-25: LABELING

Label the following image from the list of terms provided in the Chapter 6 Word List in Appendix B.

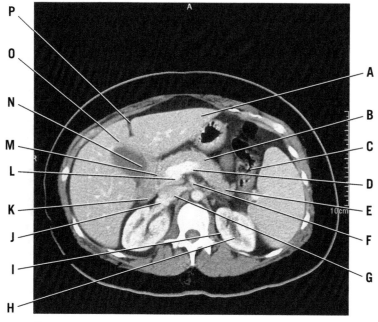

CT images provided by Our Lady of Fatima Hospital, North Providence, Rhode Island.

A. _____   I. _____

B. _____   J. _____

C. _____   K. _____

D. _____   L. _____

E. _____   M. _____

F. _____   N. _____

G. _____   O. _____

H. _____   P. _____

EXERCISE 6-26: LABELING

Label the following image from the list of terms provided in the Chapter 6 Word List in Appendix B.

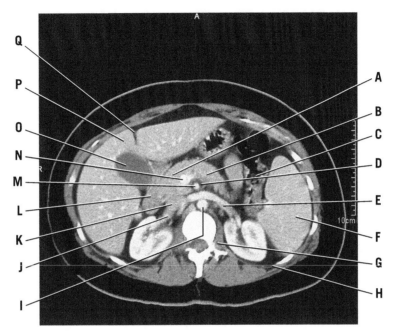

CT images provided by Our Lady of Fatima Hospital, North Providence, Rhode Island.

A. _____   J. _____

B. _____   K. _____

C. _____   L. _____

D. _____   M. _____

E. _____   N. _____

F. _____   O. _____

G. _____   P. _____

H. _____   Q. _____

I. _____

EXERCISE 6-27: LABELING

Label the following image from the list of terms provided in the Chapter 6 Word List in Appendix B.

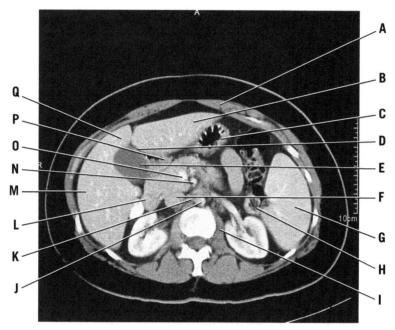

CT images provided by Our Lady of Fatima Hospital, North Providence, Rhode Island.

A. _____   J. _____

B. _____   K. _____

C. _____   L. _____

D. _____   M. _____

E. _____   N. _____

F. _____   O. _____

G. _____   P. _____

H. _____   Q. _____

I. _____

EXERCISE 6-28: LABELING

Label the following image from the list of terms provided in the Chapter 6 Word List in Appendix B.

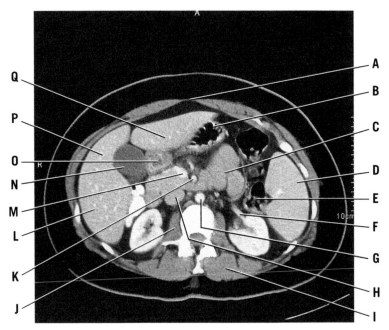

CT images provided by Our Lady of Fatima Hospital, North Providence, Rhode Island.

A. _____   J. _____

B. _____   K. _____

C. _____   L. _____

D. _____   M. _____

E. _____   N. _____

F. _____   O. _____

G. _____   P. _____

H. _____   Q. _____

I. _____

EXERCISE 6-29: LABELING

Label the following image from the list of terms provided in the Chapter 6 Word List in Appendix B.

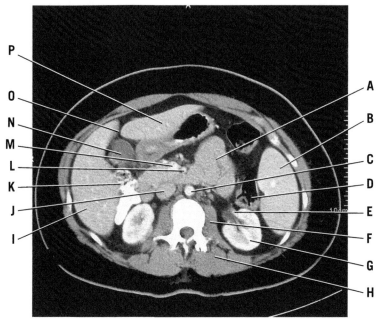

CT images provided by Our Lady of Fatima Hospital, North Providence, Rhode Island.

A. _____   I. _____

B. _____   J. _____

C. _____   K. _____

D. _____   L. _____

E. _____   M. _____

F. _____   N. _____

G. _____   O. _____

H. _____   P. _____

EXERCISE 6-30: LABELING

Label the following image from the list of terms provided in the Chapter 6 Word List in Appendix B.

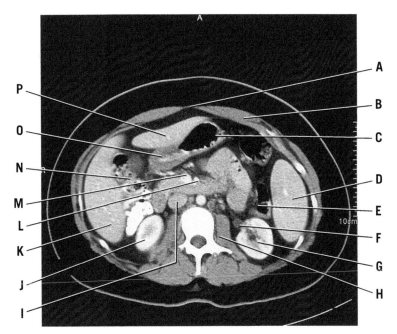

CT images provided by Our Lady of Fatima Hospital, North Providence, Rhode Island.

A. _____   I. _____

B. _____   J. _____

C. _____   K. _____

D. _____   L. _____

E. _____   M. _____

F. _____   N. _____

G. _____   O. _____

H. _____   P. _____

EXERCISE 6-31: LABELING

Label the following image from the list of terms provided in the Chapter 6 Word List in Appendix B.

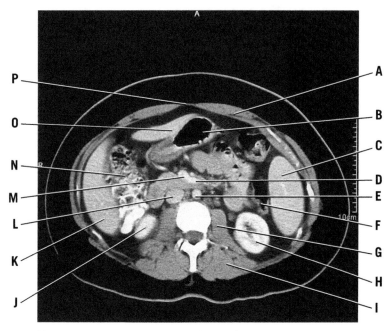

CT images provided by Our Lady of Fatima Hospital, North Providence, Rhode Island.

A. _____   I. _____

B. _____   J. _____

C. _____   K. _____

D. _____   L. _____

E. _____   M. _____

F. _____   N. _____

G. _____   O. _____

H. _____   P. _____

EXERCISE 6-32: LABELING

Label the following image from the list of terms provided in the Chapter 6 Word List in Appendix B.

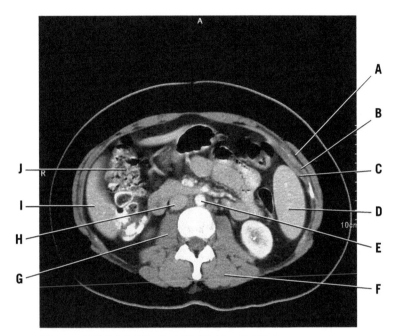

CT images provided by Our Lady of Fatima Hospital, North Providence, Rhode Island.

A. _____

B. _____

C. _____

D. _____

E. _____

F. _____

G. _____

H. _____

I. _____

J. _____

EXERCISE 6-33: LABELING

Label the following image from the list of terms provided in the Chapter 6 Word List in Appendix B.

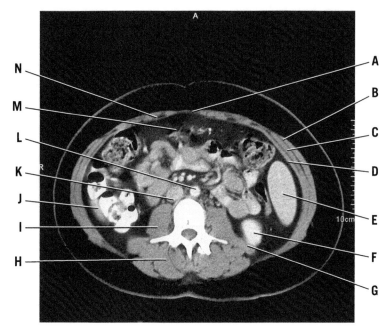

CT images provided by Our Lady of Fatima Hospital, North Providence, Rhode Island.

A. _____

B. _____

C. _____

D. _____

E. _____

F. _____

G. _____

H. _____

I. _____

J. _____

K. _____

L. _____

M. _____

N. _____

EXERCISE 6-34: LABELING

Label the following image from the list of terms provided in the Chapter 6 Word List in Appendix B.

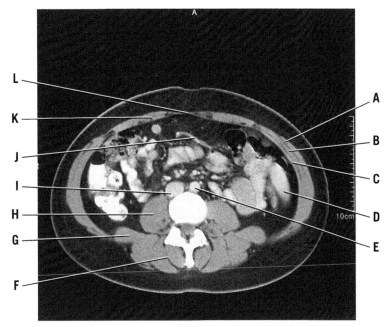

CT images provided by Our Lady of Fatima Hospital, North Providence, Rhode Island.

A. _____

B. _____

C. _____

D. _____

E. _____

F. _____

G. _____

H. _____

I. _____

J. _____

K. _____

L. _____

EXERCISE 6-35: LABELING

Label the following image from the list of terms provided in the Chapter 6 Word List in Appendix B.

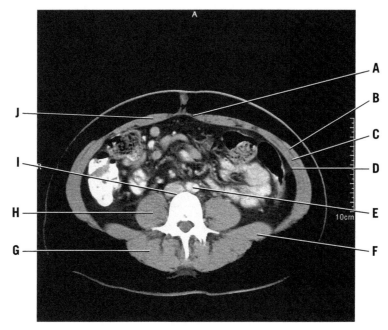

CT images provided by Our Lady of Fatima Hospital, North Providence, Rhode Island.

A. _____

B. _____

C. _____

D. _____

E. _____

F. _____

G. _____

H. _____

I. _____

J. _____

EXERCISE 6-36: LABELING

Label the following image from the list of terms provided in the Chapter 6 Word List in Appendix B.

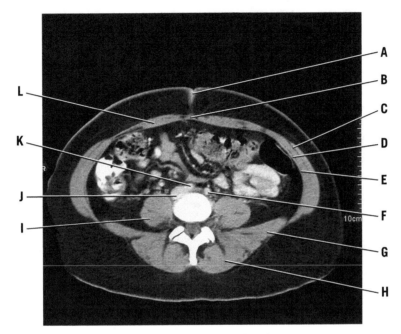

CT images provided by Our Lady of Fatima Hospital, North Providence, Rhode Island.

A. _____

B. _____

C. _____

D. _____

E. _____

F. _____

G. _____

H. _____

I. _____

J. _____

K. _____

L. _____

EXERCISE 6-37: LABELING

Label the following image from the list of terms provided in the Chapter 6 Word List in Appendix B.

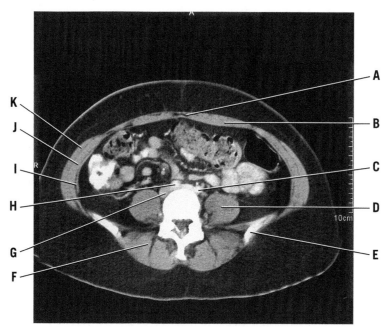

CT images provided by Our Lady of Fatima Hospital, North Providence, Rhode Island.

A. _____

B. _____

C. _____

D. _____

E. _____

F. _____

G. _____

H. _____

I. _____

J. _____

K. _____

MR IMAGES, T1 WEIGHTED

AXIAL IMAGES

EXERCISE 6-38: LABELING

Label the following image from the list of terms provided in the Chapter 6 Word List in Appendix B.

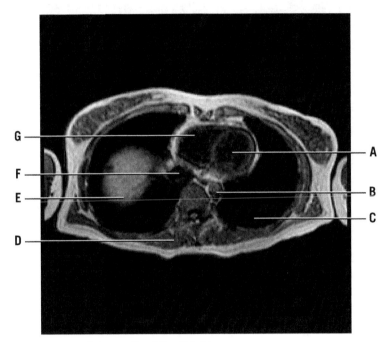

MR Images provided courtesy of Roger Williams Medical Center.

A. _____

B. _____

C. _____

D. _____

E. _____

F. _____

G. _____

EXERCISE 6-39: LABELING

Label the following image from the list of terms provided in the Chapter 6 Word List in Appendix B.

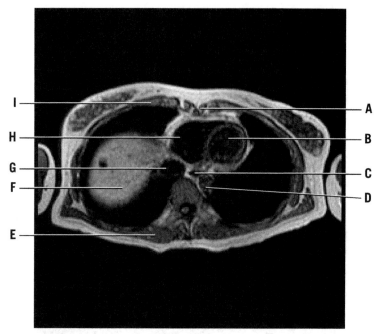

MR Images provided courtesy of Roger Williams Medical Center.

A. _____

B. _____

C. _____

D. _____

E. _____

F. _____

G. _____

H. _____

I. _____

EXERCISE 6-40: LABELING

Label the following image from the list of terms provided in the Chapter 6 Word List in Appendix B.

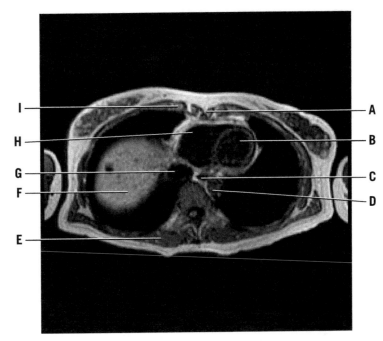

MR Images provided courtesy of Roger Williams Medical Center.

A. _____

B. _____

C. _____

D. _____

E. _____

F. _____

G. _____

H. _____

I. _____

EXERCISE 6-41: LABELING

Label the following image from the list of terms provided in the Chapter 6 Word List in Appendix B.

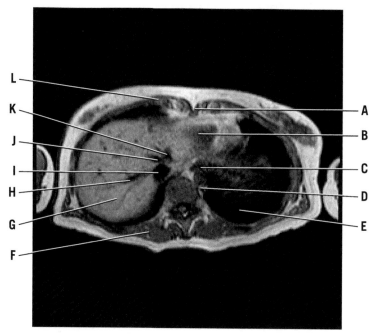

MR Images provided courtesy of Roger Williams Medical Center.

A. _____

B. _____

C. _____

D. _____

E. _____

F. _____

G. _____

H. _____

I. _____

J. _____

K. _____

L. _____

EXERCISE 6-42: LABELING

Label the following image from the list of terms provided in the Chapter 6 Word List in Appendix B.

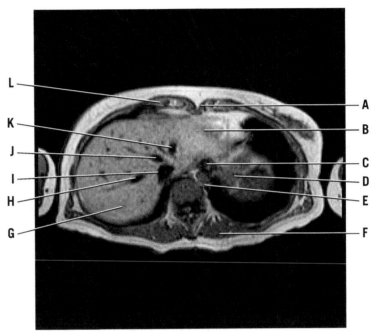

MR Images provided courtesy of Roger Williams Medical Center.

A. _____

B. _____

C. _____

D. _____

E. _____

F. _____

G. _____

H. _____

I. _____

J. _____

K. _____

L. _____

EXERCISE 6-43: LABELING

Label the following image from the list of terms provided in the Chapter 6 Word List in Appendix B.

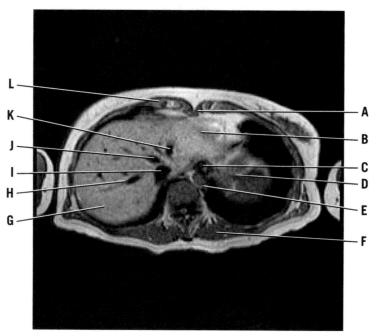

MR Images provided courtesy of Roger Williams Medical Center.

A. _____

B. _____

C. _____

D. _____

E. _____

F. _____

G. _____

H. _____

I. _____

J. _____

K. _____

L. _____

EXERCISE 6-44: LABELING

Label the following image from the list of terms provided in the Chapter 6 Word List in Appendix B.

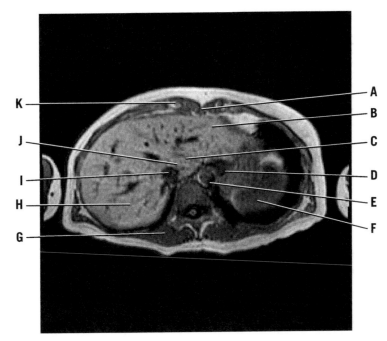

MR Images provided courtesy of Roger Williams Medical Center.

A. _____

B. _____

C. _____

D. _____

E. _____

F. _____

G. _____

H. _____

I. _____

J. _____

K. _____

EXERCISE 6-45: LABELING

Label the following image from the list of terms provided in the Chapter 6 Word List in Appendix B.

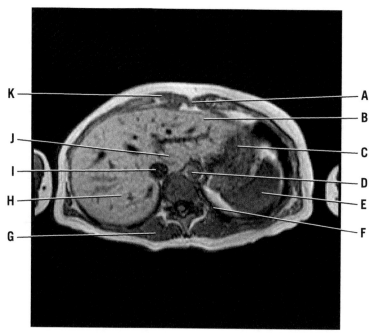

MR Images provided courtesy of Roger Williams Medical Center.

A. _____

B. _____

C. _____

D. _____

E. _____

F. _____

G. _____

H. _____

I. _____

J. _____

K. _____

EXERCISE 6-46: LABELING

Label the following image from the list of terms provided in the Chapter 6 Word List in Appendix B.

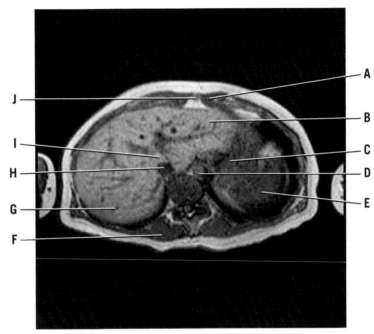

MR Images provided courtesy of Roger Williams Medical Center.

A. _____

B. _____

C. _____

D. _____

E. _____

F. _____

G. _____

H. _____

I. _____

J. _____

EXERCISE 6-47: LABELING

Label the following image from the list of terms provided in the **Chapter 6 Word List** in Appendix B.

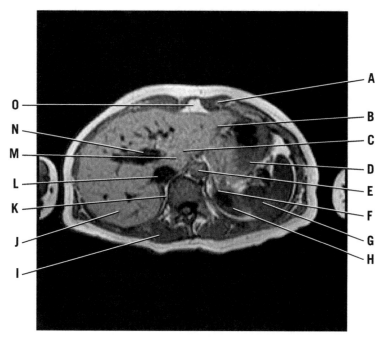

MR Images provided courtesy of Roger Williams Medical Center.

A. _____

B. _____

C. _____

D. _____

E. _____

F. _____

G. _____

H. _____

I. _____

J. _____

K. _____

L. _____

M. _____

N. _____

O. _____

EXERCISE 6-48: LABELING

Label the following image from the list of terms provided in the Chapter 6 Word List in Appendix B.

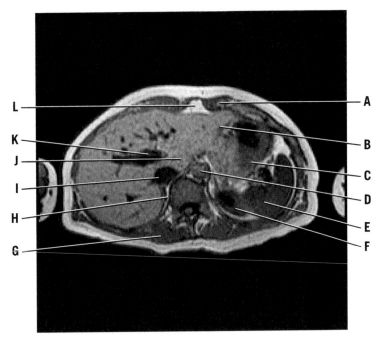

MR Images provided courtesy of Roger Williams Medical Center.

A. _____

B. _____

C. _____

D. _____

E. _____

F. _____

G. _____

H. _____

I. _____

J. _____

K. _____

L. _____

EXERCISE 6-49: LABELING

Label the following image from the list of terms provided in the Chapter 6 Word List in Appendix B.

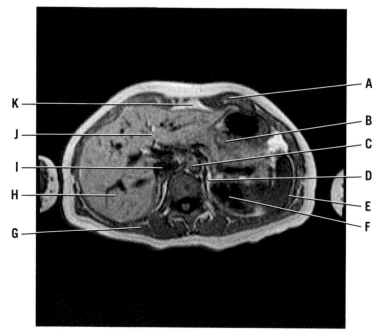

MR Images provided courtesy of Roger Williams Medical Center.

A. _____

B. _____

C. _____

D. _____

E. _____

F. _____

G. _____

H. _____

I. _____

J. _____

K. _____

EXERCISE 6-50: LABELING

Label the following image from the list of terms provided in the Chapter 6 Word List in Appendix B.

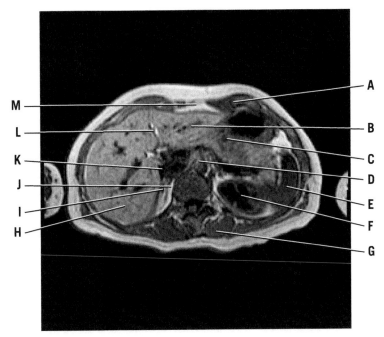

MR Images provided courtesy of Roger Williams Medical Center.

A. _____

B. _____

C. _____

D. _____

E. _____

F. _____

G. _____

H. _____

I. _____

J. _____

K. _____

L. _____

M. _____

EXERCISE 6-51: LABELING

Label the following image from the list of terms provided in the Chapter 6 Word List in Appendix B.

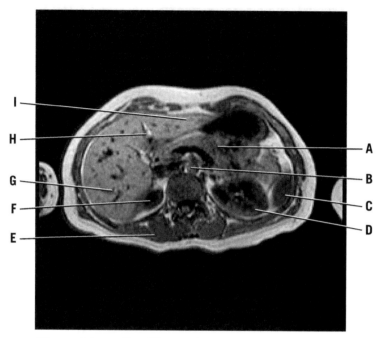

MR Images provided courtesy of Roger Williams Medical Center.

A. _____

B. _____

C. _____

D. _____

E. _____

F. _____

G. _____

H. _____

I. _____

EXERCISE 6-52: LABELING

Label the following image from the list of terms provided in the Chapter 6 Word List in Appendix B.

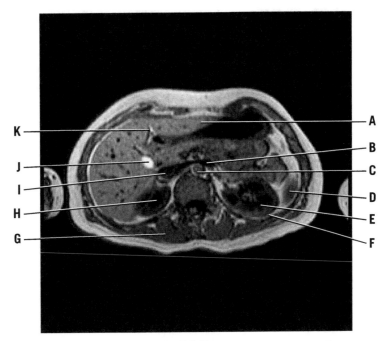

MR Images provided courtesy of Roger Williams Medical Center.

A. _____

B. _____

C. _____

D. _____

E. _____

F. _____

G. _____

H. _____

I. _____

J. _____

K. _____

EXERCISE 6-53: LABELING

Label the following image from the list of terms provided in the Chapter 6 Word List in Appendix B.

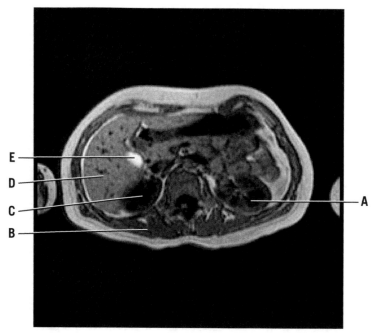

MR Images provided courtesy of Roger Williams Medical Center.

A. _____

B. _____

C. _____

D. _____

E. _____

EXERCISE 6-54: LABELING

Label the following image from the list of terms provided in the Chapter 6 Word List in Appendix B.

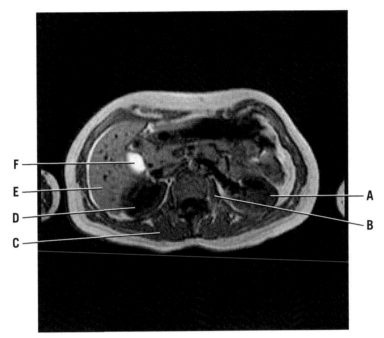

MR Images provided courtesy of Roger Williams Medical Center.

A. _____

B. _____

C. _____

D. _____

E. _____

F. _____

EXERCISE 6-55: LABELING

Label the following image from the list of terms provided in the Chapter 6 Word List in Appendix B.

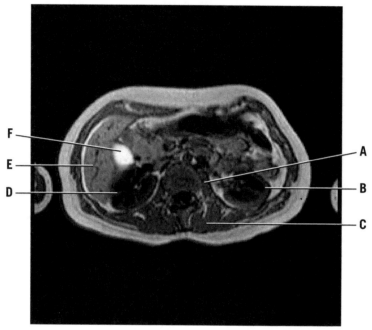

MR Images provided courtesy of Roger Williams Medical Center.

A. _____

B. _____

C. _____

D. _____

E. _____

F. _____

EXERCISE 6-56: LABELING

Label the following image from the list of terms provided in the Chapter 6 Word List in Appendix B.

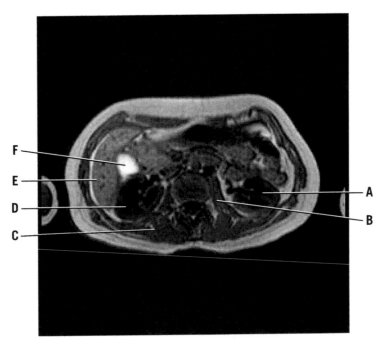

MR Images provided courtesy of Roger Williams Medical Center.

A. _____

B. _____

C. _____

D. _____

E. _____

F. _____

EXERCISE 6-57: LABELING

Label the following image from the list of terms provided in the Chapter 6 Word List in Appendix B.

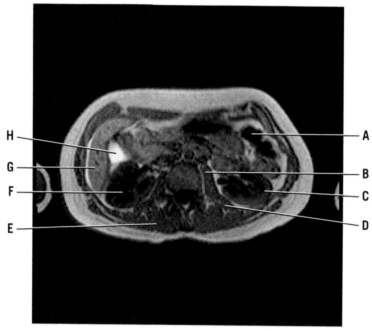

MR Images provided courtesy of Roger Williams Medical Center.

A. _____

B. _____

C. _____

D. _____

E. _____

F. _____

G. _____

H. _____

EXERCISE 6-58: LABELING

Label the following image from the list of terms provided in the Chapter 6 Word List in Appendix B.

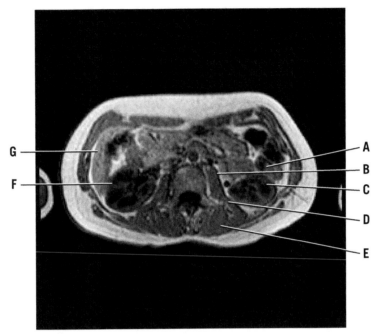

MR Images provided courtesy of Roger Williams Medical Center.

A. _____

B. _____

C. _____

D. _____

E. _____

F. _____

G. _____

EXERCISE 6-59: LABELING

Label the following image from the list of terms provided in the Chapter 6 Word List in Appendix B.

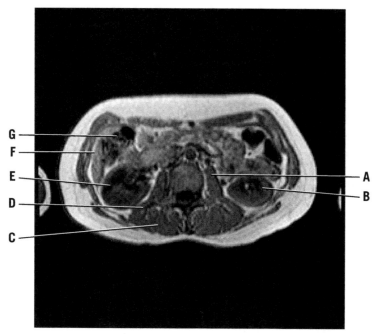

MR Images provided courtesy of Roger Williams Medical Center.

A. _____

B. _____

C. _____

D. _____

E. _____

F. _____

G. _____

EXERCISE 6-60: LABELING

Label the following image from the list of terms provided in the Chapter 6 Word List in Appendix B.

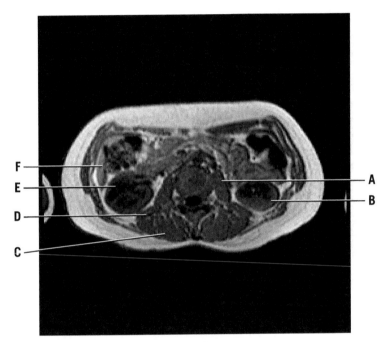

MR Images provided courtesy of Roger Williams Medical Center.

A. _____

B. _____

C. _____

D. _____

E. _____

F. _____

EXERCISE 6-61: LABELING

Label the following image from the list of terms provided in the Chapter 6 Word List in Appendix B.

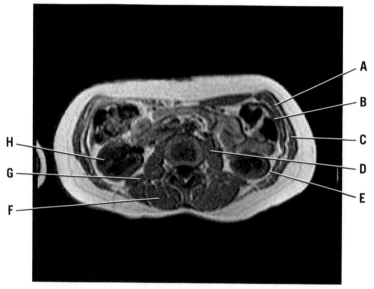

MR Images provided courtesy of Roger Williams Medical Center.

A. _____

B. _____

C. _____

D. _____

E. _____

F. _____

G. _____

H. _____

EXERCISE 6-62: LABELING

Label the following image from the list of terms provided in the Chapter 6 Word List in Appendix B.

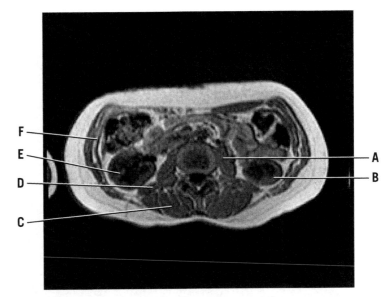

F
E
D
C
A
B

MR Images provided courtesy of Roger Williams Medical Center.

A. _____

B. _____

C. _____

D. _____

E. _____

F. _____

EXERCISE 6-63: LABELING

Label the following image from the list of terms provided in the Chapter 6 Word List in Appendix B.

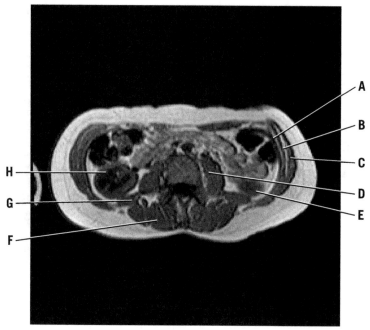

MR Images provided courtesy of Roger Williams Medical Center.

A. _____

B. _____

C. _____

D. _____

E. _____

F. _____

G. _____

H. _____

EXERCISE 6-64: LABELING

Label the following image from the list of terms provided in the Chapter 6 Word List in Appendix B.

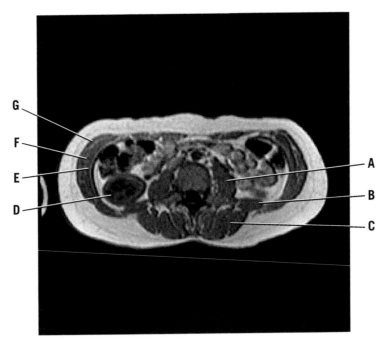

MR Images provided courtesy of Roger Williams Medical Center.

A. _____

B. _____

C. _____

D. _____

E. _____

F. _____

G. _____

EXERCISE 6-65: LABELING

Label the following image from the list of terms provided in the Chapter 6 Word List in Appendix B.

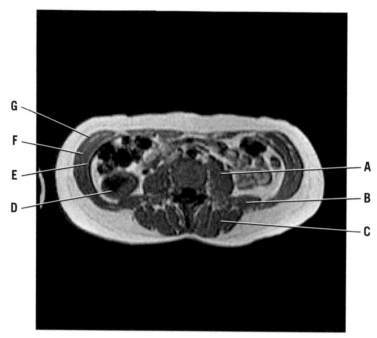

MR Images provided courtesy of Roger Williams Medical Center.

A. _____

B. _____

C. _____

D. _____

E. _____

F. _____

G. _____

EXERCISE 6-66: LABELING

Label the following image from the list of terms provided in the Chapter 6 Word List in Appendix B.

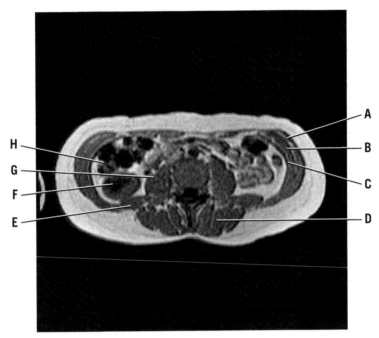

MR Images provided courtesy of Roger Williams Medical Center.

A. _____

B. _____

C. _____

D. _____

E. _____

F. _____

G. _____

H. _____

EXERCISE 6-67: LABELING

Label the following image from the list of terms provided in the Chapter 6 Word List in Appendix B.

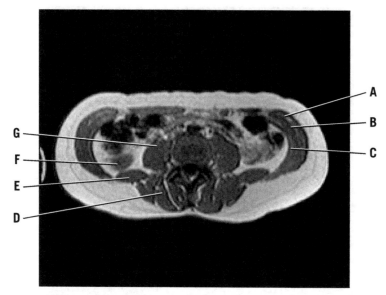

MR Images provided courtesy of Roger Williams Medical Center.

A. _____

B. _____

C. _____

D. _____

E. _____

F. _____

G. _____

EXERCISE 6-68: LABELING

Label the following image from the list of terms provided in the Chapter 6 Word List in Appendix B.

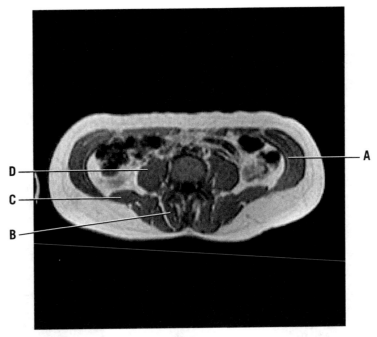

MR Images provided courtesy of Roger Williams Medical Center.

A. _____

B. _____

C. _____

D. _____

CORONAL IMAGES

EXERCISE 6-69: LABELING

Label the following image from the list of terms provided in the Chapter 6 Word List in Appendix B.

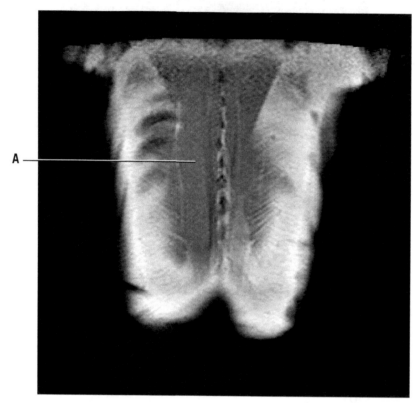

MR Images provided courtesy of Roger Williams Medical Center.

A. _____

EXERCISE 6-70: LABELING

Label the following image from the list of terms provided in the Chapter 6 Word List in Appendix B.

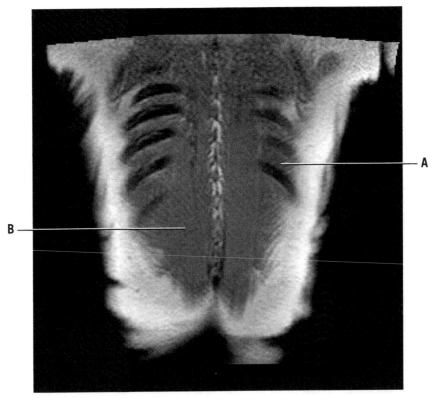

MR Images provided courtesy of Roger Williams Medical Center.

A. _____

B. _____

EXERCISE 6-71: LABELING

Label the following image from the list of terms provided in the Chapter 6 Word List in Appendix B.

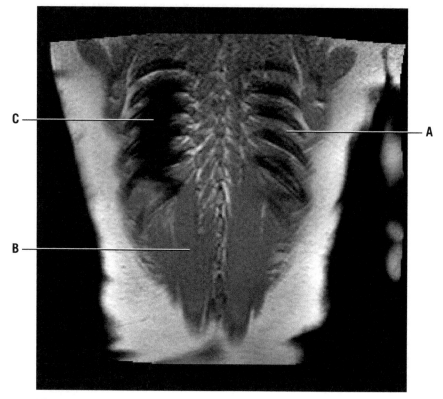

C —

B —

— A

MR Images provided courtesy of Roger Williams Medical Center.

A. _____

B. _____

C. _____

EXERCISE 6-72: LABELING

Label the following image from the list of terms provided in the Chapter 6 Word List in Appendix B.

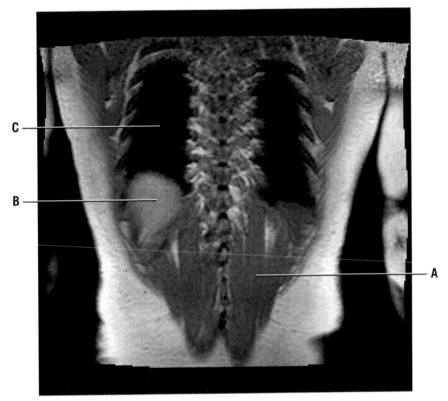

MR Images provided courtesy of Roger Williams Medical Center.

A. _____

B. _____

C. _____

EXERCISE 6-73: LABELING

Label the following image from the list of terms provided in the Chapter 6 Word List in Appendix B.

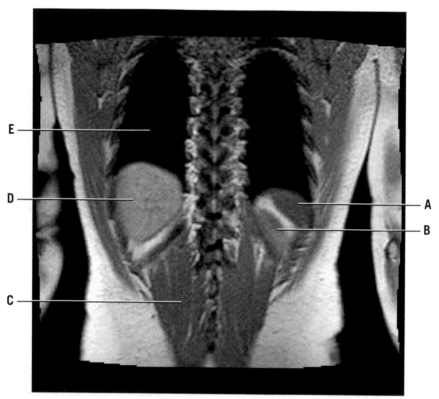

MR Images provided courtesy of Roger Williams Medical Center.

A. _____

B. _____

C. _____

D. _____

E. _____

EXERCISE 6-74: LABELING

Label the following image from the list of terms provided in the Chapter 6 Word List in Appendix B.

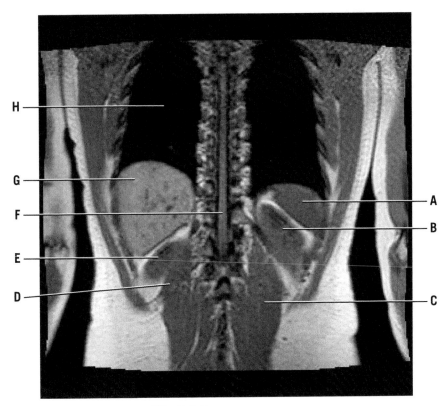

MR Images provided courtesy of Roger Williams Medical Center.

A. _____

B. _____

C. _____

D. _____

E. _____

F. _____

G. _____

H. _____

EXERCISE 6-75: LABELING

Label the following image from the list of terms provided in the Chapter 6 Word List in Appendix B.

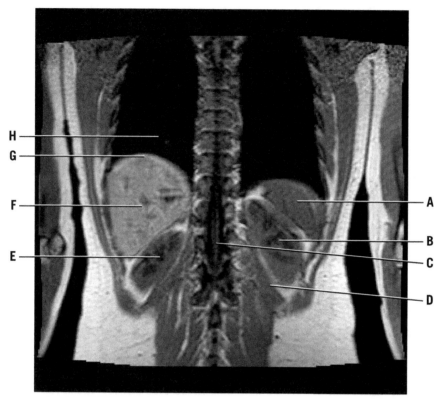

MR Images provided courtesy of Roger Williams Medical Center.

A. _____

B. _____

C. _____

D. _____

E. _____

F. _____

G. _____

H. _____

EXERCISE 6-76: LABELING

Label the following image from the list of terms provided in the Chapter 6 Word List in Appendix B.

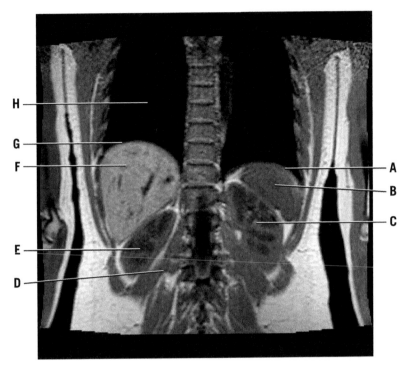

MR Images provided courtesy of Roger Williams Medical Center.

A. _____

B. _____

C. _____

D. _____

E. _____

F. _____

G. _____

H. _____

EXERCISE 6-77: LABELING

Label the following image from the list of terms provided in the Chapter 6 Word List in Appendix B.

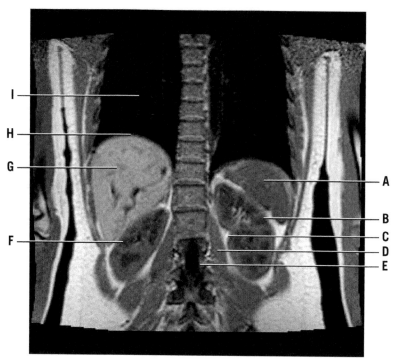

MR Images provided courtesy of Roger Williams Medical Center.

A. _____

B. _____

C. _____

D. _____

E. _____

F. _____

G. _____

H. _____

I. _____

EXERCISE 6-78: LABELING

Label the following image from the list of terms provided in the Chapter 6 Word List in Appendix B.

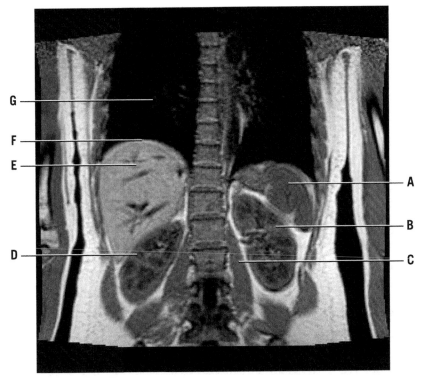

MR Images provided courtesy of Roger Williams Medical Center.

A. _____

B. _____

C. _____

D. _____

E. _____

F. _____

G. _____

EXERCISE 6-79: LABELING

Label the following image from the list of terms provided in the **Chapter 6 Word List** in Appendix B.

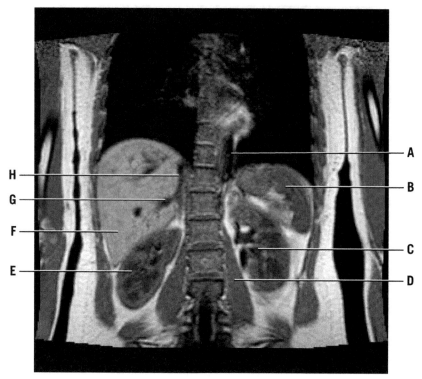

MR Images provided courtesy of Roger Williams Medical Center.

A. _____

B. _____

C. _____

D. _____

E. _____

F. _____

G. _____

H. _____

EXERCISE 6-80: LABELING

Label the following image from the list of terms provided in the Chapter 6 Word List in Appendix B.

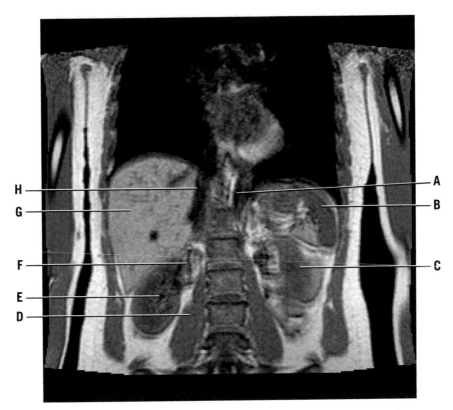

MR Images provided courtesy of Roger Williams Medical Center.

A. _____

B. _____

C. _____

D. _____

E. _____

F. _____

G. _____

H. _____

EXERCISE 6-81: LABELING

Label the following image from the list of terms provided in the Chapter 6 Word List in Appendix B.

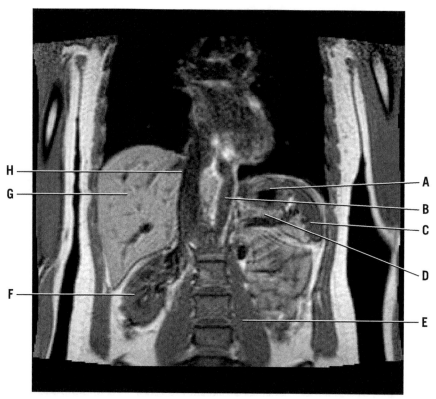

MR Images provided courtesy of Roger Williams Medical Center.

A. _____

B. _____

C. _____

D. _____

E. _____

F. _____

G. _____

H. _____

EXERCISE 6-82: LABELING

Label the following image from the list of terms provided in the Chapter 6 Word List in Appendix B.

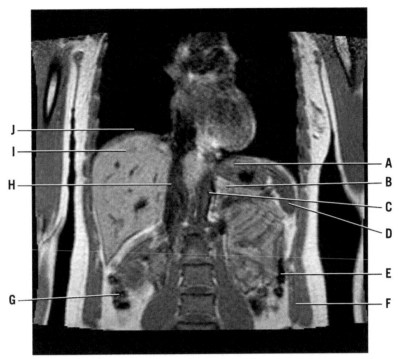

MR Images provided courtesy of Roger Williams Medical Center.

A. _____

B. _____

C. _____

D. _____

E. _____

F. _____

G. _____

H. _____

I. _____

J. _____

EXERCISE 6-83: LABELING

Label the following image from the list of terms provided in the Chapter 6 Word List in Appendix B.

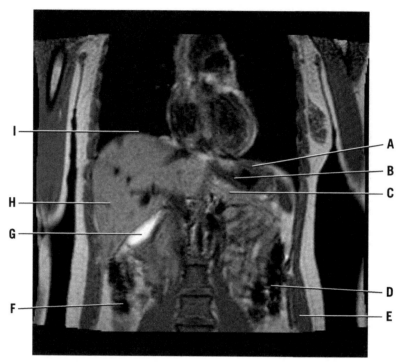

MR Images provided courtesy of Roger Williams Medical Center.

A. _____

B. _____

C. _____

D. _____

E. _____

F. _____

G. _____

H. _____

I. _____

EXERCISE 6-84: LABELING

Label the following image from the list of terms provided in the Chapter 6 Word List in Appendix B.

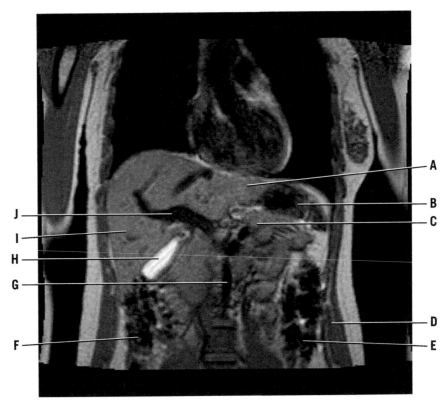

MR Images provided courtesy of Roger Williams Medical Center.

A. _____

B. _____

C. _____

D. _____

E. _____

F. _____

G. _____

H. _____

I. _____

J. _____

EXERCISE 6-85: LABELING

Label the following image from the list of terms provided in the Chapter 6 Word List in Appendix B.

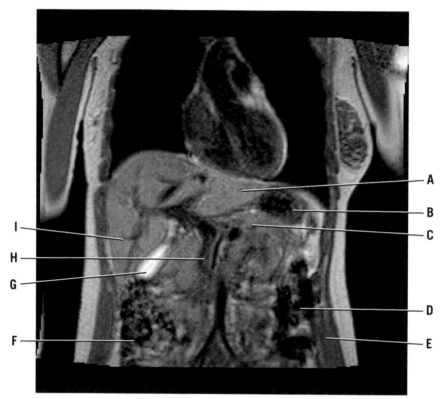

MR Images provided courtesy of Roger Williams Medical Center.

A. _____

B. _____

C. _____

D. _____

E. _____

F. _____

G. _____

H. _____

I. _____

EXERCISE 6-86: LABELING

Label the following image from the list of terms provided in the Chapter 6 Word List in Appendix B.

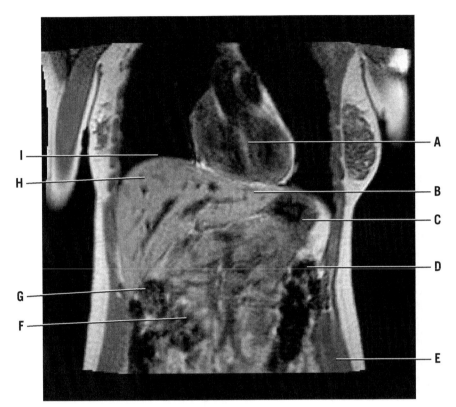

MR Images provided courtesy of Roger Williams Medical Center.

A. _____

B. _____

C. _____

D. _____

E. _____

F. _____

G. _____

H. _____

I. _____

EXERCISE 6-87: LABELING

Label the following image from the list of terms provided in the Chapter 6 Word List in Appendix B.

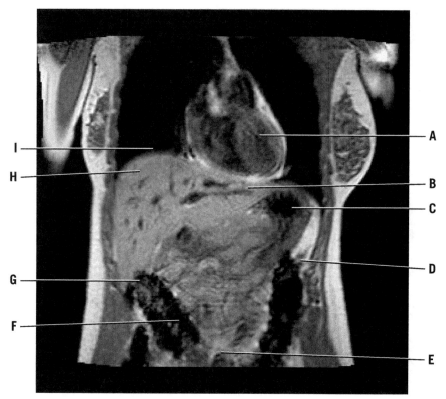

MR Images provided courtesy of Roger Williams Medical Center.

A. _____

B. _____

C. _____

D. _____

E. _____

F. _____

G. _____

H. _____

I. _____

EXERCISE 6-88: LABELING

Label the following image from the list of terms provided in the Chapter 6 Word List in Appendix B.

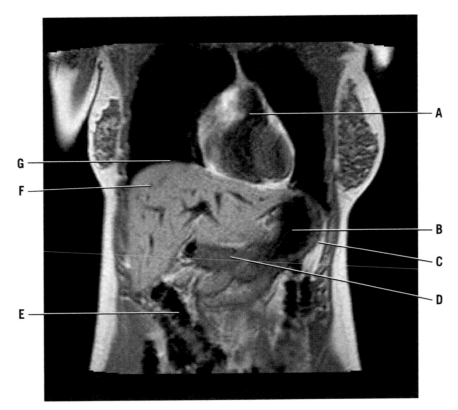

MR Images provided courtesy of Roger Williams Medical Center.

A. _____

B. _____

C. _____

D. _____

E. _____

F. _____

G. _____

EXERCISE 6-89: LABELING

Label the following image from the list of terms provided in the Chapter 6 Word List in Appendix B.

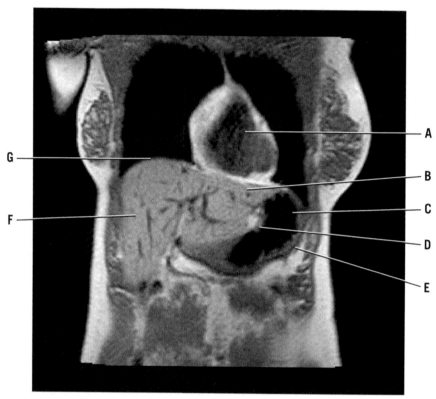

MR Images provided courtesy of Roger Williams Medical Center.

A. _____

B. _____

C. _____

D. _____

E. _____

F. _____

G. _____

EXERCISE 6-90: LABELING

Label the following image from the list of terms provided in the Chapter 6 Word List in Appendix B.

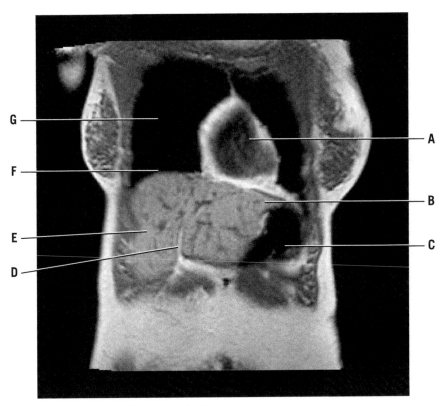

MR Images provided courtesy of Roger Williams Medical Center.

A. _____

B. _____

C. _____

D. _____

E. _____

F. _____

G. _____

EXERCISE 6-91: LABELING

Label the following image from the list of terms provided in the Chapter 6 Word List in Appendix B.

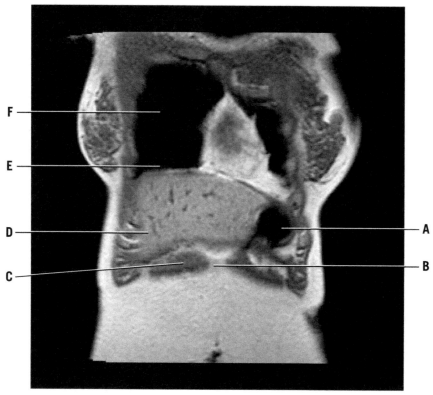

MR Images provided courtesy of Roger Williams Medical Center.

A. _____

B. _____

C. _____

D. _____

E. _____

F. _____

EXERCISE 6-92: LABELING

Label the following image from the list of terms provided in the Chapter 6 Word List in Appendix B.

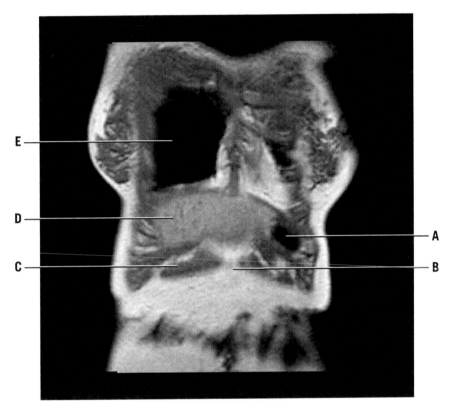

MR Images provided courtesy of Roger Williams Medical Center.

A. _____

B. _____

C. _____

D. _____

E. _____

EXERCISE 6-93: LABELING

Label the following image from the list of terms provided in the Chapter 6 Word List in Appendix B.

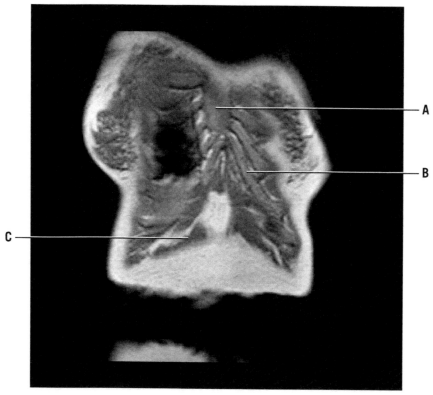

MR Images provided courtesy of Roger Williams Medical Center.

A. _____

B. _____

C. _____

Pelvis

OUTLINE

EXERCISE 7-1: COMPLETION

Complete the following by selecting the correct term from the list provided.

bulbourethral glands   ejaculatory duct   prostate gland   seminal vesicles
Cowper's glands   epididymis   scrotum   testicles
ductus vas deferens   prostatic urethra   seminal vesicle duct   testis

Sperm is manufactured in the _____ or _____.
Once produced, they mature in the _____. After leaving the
_____, they pass through the _____, which ascends
along the anterior bladder and then passes along the lateral bladder, descending posterior to the
bladder. Two structures that produce approximately 60 percent of the seminal fluid are located
on either side of the posterior bladder, the _____. The fluid manufactured
by them passes into the _____, forming a new passageway at the base
of the bladder, the _____. These bilateral vessels empty into the single
_____, which has the _____ encircling it. The function
of the _____ is to prevent the mix of urine and semen and to produce some
of the seminal fluid. The _____ is the largest accessory gland of the male
reproductive system. Inferior to this are two pea-size organs, the _____ or
_____. They also contribute to the seminal fluid and lubricate the end of the
penis during intercourse.

EXERCISE 7-2: IDENTIFICATION

Identify the three main parts of the uterus.

1. _____
2. _____
3. _____

EXERCISE 7-3: MATCHING

Match the following terms with the correct definitions.

_____ 1. cervix

_____ 2. fimbria

_____ 3. fornix

_____ 4. infundibulum

_____ 5. ovaries

_____ 6. vagina

a. lateral end of the uterine or fallopian tube

b. paired sex glands in the female producing the female egg and female hormones

c. one of many fingerlike processes extending from the infundibulum of the uterine tube resembling a fringe

d. passageway in females for penile insertion during coitus, delivery of infant at end of pregnancy, and flow of blood during menstruation

e. narrowed inferior portion of the uterus that leads to the vagina

f. archlike structure; the recess where the cervix meets the vagina

EXERCISE 7-4: SORTING

Number the gluteal muscles in the order that they appear on axial CT images arranged in descending order.

_____ 1. gluteal maximus

_____ 2. gluteal medius

_____ 3. gluteal minimus

EXERCISE 7-5: MATCHING

Match the following muscles with the definitions that best describe them.

_____ 1. gluteal muscles

_____ 2. levator ani

_____ 3. pectineus

_____ 4. piriformis

_____ 5. rectus abdominis

_____ 6. sartorius

a. longest muscle in the human body

b. lateral to the pubic rami

c. involved in forming the pelvic floor

d. posterolateral pelvic region

e. anterior abdomen

f. anterior to the sacrum

EXERCISE 7-6: MATCHING

Match the following terms with the correct definitions.

____ 1. acetabulum

____ 2. ala

____ 3. Cowper's gland

____ 4. false pelvis

____ 5. genitalia

____ 6. infundibulum

____ 7. oviduct

____ 8. ovum

____ 9. pudendum

____ 10. seminal vesical

a. the cavity found above and anterior to the pelvic inlet

b. the lateral end of the uterine or fallopian tube

c. a wing-shaped structure

d. a mature female egg or germ cell produced by the ovaries

e. the cup-shaped lateral portion of the innominate bone articulating with the head of the femur

f. external female genitalia

g. a bilateral gland in males found behind the bladder producing a large percentage of seminal fluid

h. a bilateral accessory reproductive gland in the male located on either side of the prostate gland producing a small amount of seminal fluid

i. reproductive or sex organs

j. a bilateral tube extending laterally from the uterus that serves as a site for fertilization of a female ovum or egg by the male sperm

EXERCISE 7-7: LABELING

Label the following illustration from the list of terms provided.

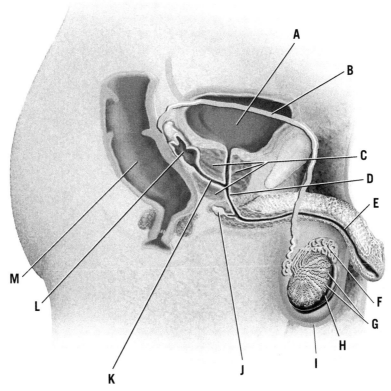

Copyright © 2015 Cengage Learning®.

bulbourethral gland
ductus vas deferens
ejaculatory duct
epididymis
prostate gland
prostatic urethra
rectum
scrotum
seminal vesicle
seminiferous tubules
testis
urethra
urinary bladder

A. _____

B. _____

C. _____

D. _____

E. _____

F. _____

G. _____

H. _____

I. _____

J. _____

K. _____

L. _____

M. _____

EXERCISE 7-8: LABELING

Label the following illustration from the list of terms provided.

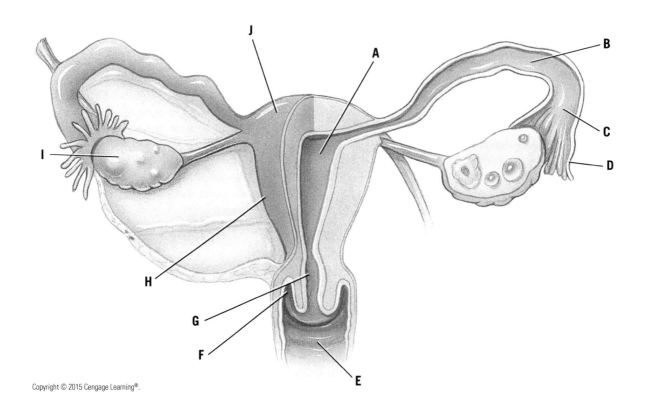

Copyright © 2015 Cengage Learning®.

body of uterus
cervix of uterus
fimbriae
fornix
fundus of uterus
infundibulum
ovary
uterine cavity
uterine tube
vagina

A. _____

B. _____

C. _____

D. _____

E. _____

F. _____

G. _____

H. _____

I. _____

J. _____

CT AXIAL IMAGES

EXERCISE 7-9: LABELING

Label the following image from the list of terms provided in the **Chapter 7 Word List** in Appendix B.

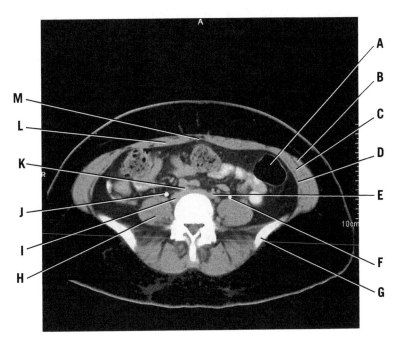

CT images provided by Our Lady of Fatima Hospital, North Providence, Rhode Island.

A. _____

B. _____

C. _____

D. _____

E. _____

F. _____

G. _____

H. _____

I. _____

J. _____

K. _____

L. _____

M. _____

EXERCISE 7-10: LABELING

Label the following image from the list of terms provided in the Chapter 7 Word List in Appendix B.

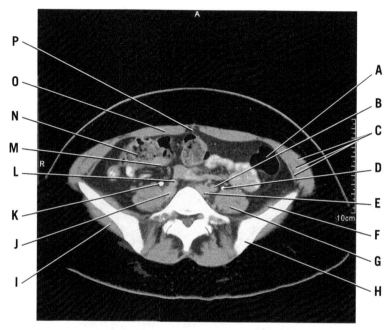

CT images provided by Our Lady of Fatima Hospital, North Providence, Rhode Island.

A. _____   I. _____

B. _____   J. _____

C. _____   K. _____

D. _____   L. _____

E. _____   M. _____

F. _____   N. _____

G. _____   O. _____

H. _____   P. _____

EXERCISE 7-11: LABELING

Label the following image from the list of terms provided in the Chapter 7 Word List in Appendix B.

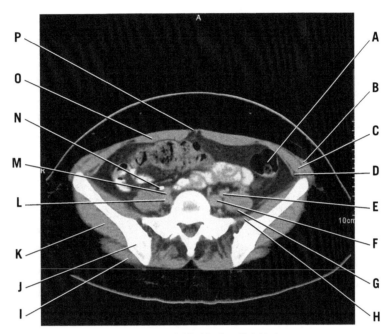

CT images provided by Our Lady of Fatima Hospital, North Providence, Rhode Island.

A. _____

B. _____

C. _____

D. _____

E. _____

F. _____

G. _____

H. _____

I. _____

J. _____

K. _____

L. _____

M. _____

N. _____

O. _____

P. _____

EXERCISE 7-12: LABELING

Label the following image from the list of terms provided in the Chapter 7 Word List in Appendix B.

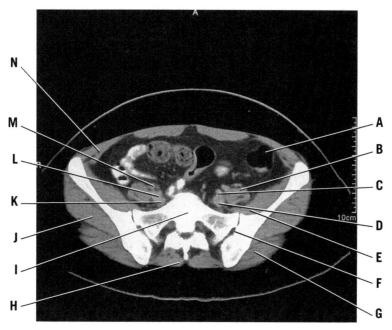

CT images provided by Our Lady of Fatima Hospital, North Providence, Rhode Island.

A. _____

B. _____

C. _____

D. _____

E. _____

F. _____

G. _____

H. _____

I. _____

J. _____

K. _____

L. _____

M. _____

N. _____

EXERCISE 7-13: LABELING

Label the following image from the list of terms provided in the Chapter 7 Word List in Appendix B.

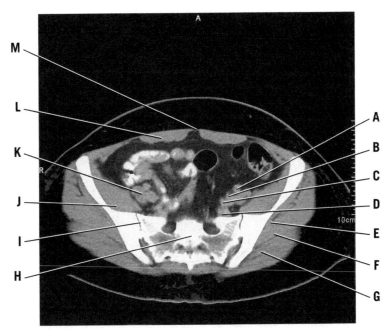

CT images provided by Our Lady of Fatima Hospital, North Providence, Rhode Island.

A. _____

B. _____

C. _____

D. _____

E. _____

F. _____

G. _____

H. _____

I. _____

J. _____

K. _____

L. _____

M. _____

EXERCISE 7-14: LABELING

Label the following image from the list of terms provided in the Chapter 7 Word List in Appendix B.

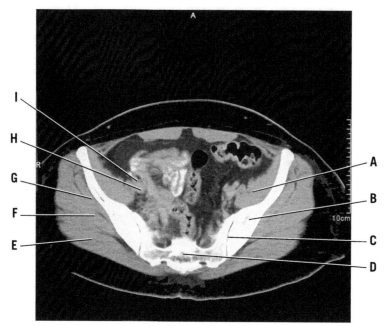

CT images provided by Our Lady of Fatima Hospital, North Providence, Rhode Island.

A. _____

B. _____

C. _____

D. _____

E. _____

F. _____

G. _____

H. _____

I. _____

EXERCISE 7-15: LABELING

Label the following image from the list of terms provided in the Chapter 7 Word List in Appendix B.

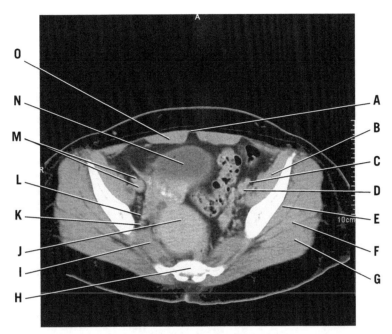

CT images provided by Our Lady of Fatima Hospital, North Providence, Rhode Island.

A. _____

B. _____

C. _____

D. _____

E. _____

F. _____

G. _____

H. _____

I. _____

J. _____

K. _____

L. _____

M. _____

N. _____

O. _____

EXERCISE 7-16: LABELING

Label the following image from the list of terms provided in the Chapter 7 Word List in Appendix B.

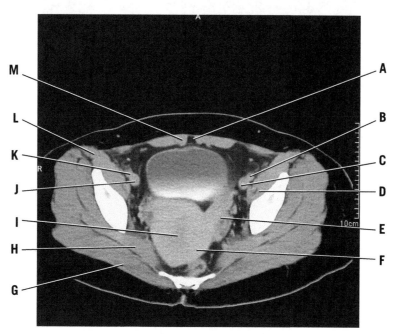

CT images provided by Our Lady of Fatima Hospital, North Providence, Rhode Island.

A. _____

B. _____

C. _____

D. _____

E. _____

F. _____

G. _____

H. _____

I. _____

J. _____

K. _____

L. _____

M. _____

EXERCISE 7-17: LABELING

Label the following image from the list of terms provided in the Chapter 7 Word List in Appendix B.

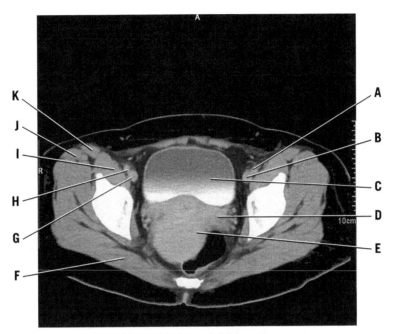

CT Images provided by Our Lady of Fatima Hospital, North Providence, Rhode Island

A. _____

B. _____

C. _____

D. _____

E. _____

F. _____

G. _____

H. _____

I. _____

J. _____

K. _____

EXERCISE 7-18: LABELING

Label the following image from the list of terms provided in the Chapter 7 Word List in Appendix B.

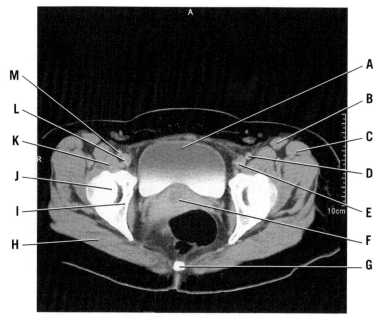

CT Images provided by Our Lady of Fatima Hospital, North Providence, Rhode Island

A. _____

B. _____

C. _____

D. _____

E. _____

F. _____

G. _____

H. _____

I. _____

J. _____

K. _____

L. _____

M. _____

EXERCISE 7-19: LABELING

Label the following image from the list of terms provided in the Chapter 7 Word List in Appendix B.

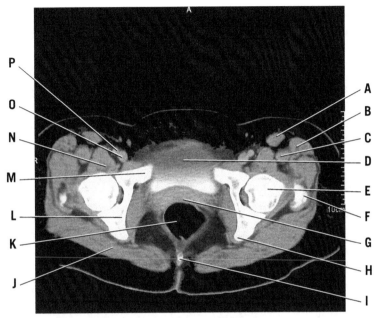

CT Images provided by Our Lady of Fatima Hospital, North Providence, Rhode Island

A. _____   I. _____

B. _____   J. _____

C. _____   K. _____

D. _____   L. _____

E. _____   M. _____

F. _____   N. _____

G. _____   O. _____

H. _____   P. _____

EXERCISE 7-20: LABELING

Label the following image from the list of terms provided in the Chapter 7 Word List in Appendix B.

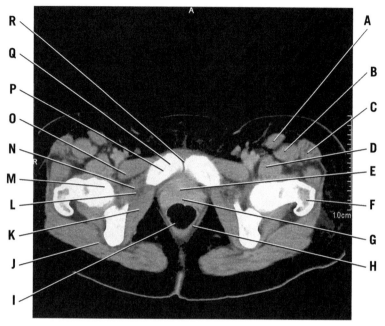

CT Images provided by Our Lady of Fatima Hospital, North Providence, Rhode Island

A. _____   J. _____

B. _____   K. _____

C. _____   L. _____

D. _____   M. _____

E. _____   N. _____

F. _____   O. _____

G. _____   P. _____

H. _____   Q. _____

I. _____   R. _____

EXERCISE 7-21: LABELING

Label the following image from the list of terms provided in the Chapter 7 Word List in Appendix B.

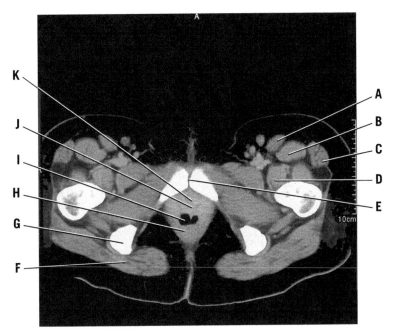

CT Images provided by Our Lady of Fatima Hospital, North Providence, Rhode Island

A. _____

B. _____

C. _____

D. _____

E. _____

F. _____

G. _____

H. _____

I. _____

J. _____

K. _____

EXERCISE 7-22: LABELING

Label the following image from the list of terms provided in the Chapter 7 Word List in Appendix B.

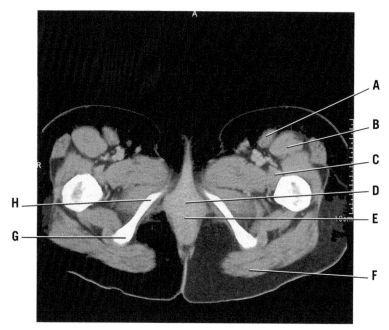

CT Images provided by Our Lady of Fatima Hospital, North Providence, Rhode Island

A. _____

B. _____

C. _____

D. _____

E. _____

F. _____

G. _____

H. _____

MR IMAGES, T2 WEIGHTED

AXIAL IMAGES OF A FEMALE PELVIS

EXERCISE 7-23: LABELING

Label the following image from the list of terms provided in the Chapter 7 Word List in Appendix B.

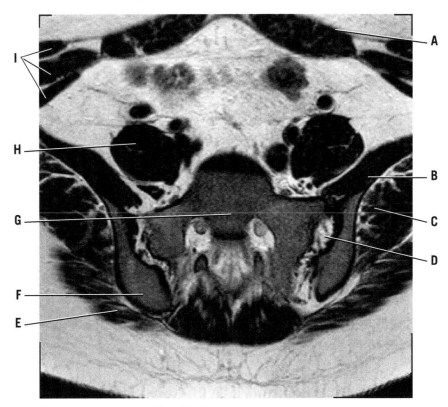

MR images provided courtesy of Roger Williams Medical Center.

A. _____

B. _____

C. _____

D. _____

E. _____

F. _____

G. _____

H. _____

I. _____

EXERCISE 7-24: LABELING

Label the following image from the list of terms provided in the Chapter 7 Word List in Appendix B.

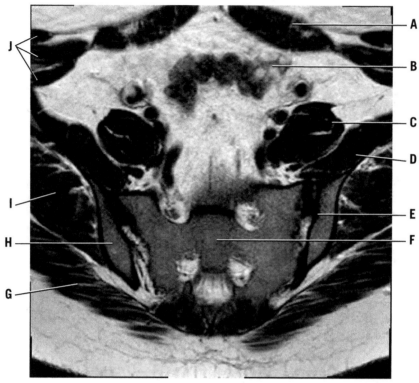

MR images provided courtesy of Roger Williams Medical Center.

A. _____

B. _____

C. _____

D. _____

E. _____

F. _____

G. _____

H. _____

I. _____

J. _____

EXERCISE 7-25: LABELING

Label the following image from the list of terms provided in the Chapter 7 Word List in Appendix B.

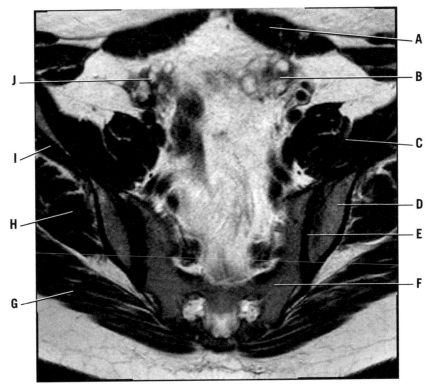

MR images provided courtesy of Roger Williams Medical Center.

A. _____

B. _____

C. _____

D. _____

E. _____

F. _____

G. _____

H. _____

I. _____

J. _____

EXERCISE 7-26: LABELING

Label the following image from the list of terms provided in the Chapter 7 Word List in Appendix B.

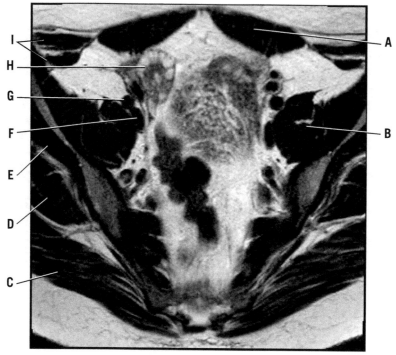

MR images provided courtesy of Roger Williams Medical Center.

A. _____

B. _____

C. _____

D. _____

E. _____

F. _____

G. _____

H. _____

I. _____

EXERCISE 7-27: LABELING

Label the following image from the list of terms provided in the Chapter 7 Word List in Appendix B.

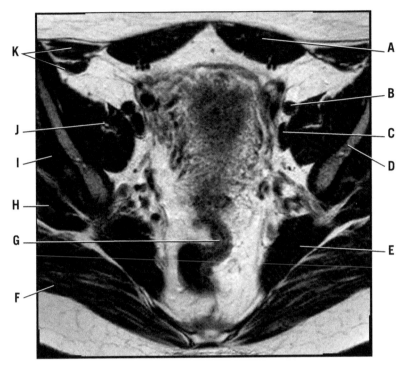

MR images provided courtesy of Roger Williams Medical Center.

A. _____

B. _____

C. _____

D. _____

E. _____

F. _____

G. _____

H. _____

I. _____

J. _____

K. _____

EXERCISE 7-28: LABELING

Label the following image from the list of terms provided in the Chapter 7 Word List in Appendix B.

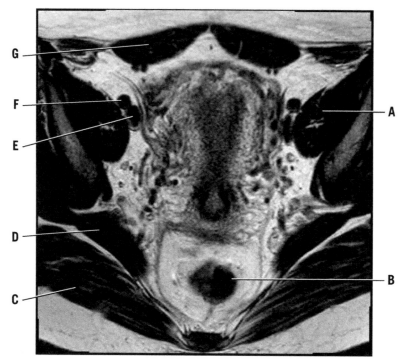

MR images provided courtesy of Roger Williams Medical Center.

A. _____

B. _____

C. _____

D. _____

E. _____

F. _____

G. _____

EXERCISE 7-29: LABELING

Label the following image from the list of terms provided in the Chapter 7 Word List in Appendix B.

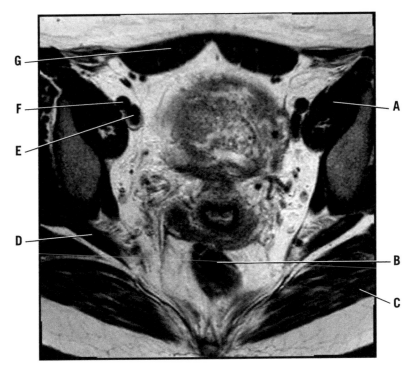

MR images provided courtesy of Roger Williams Medical Center.

A. _____

B. _____

C. _____

D. _____

E. _____

F. _____

G. _____

EXERCISE 7-30: LABELING

Label the following image from the list of terms provided in the Chapter 7 Word List in Appendix B.

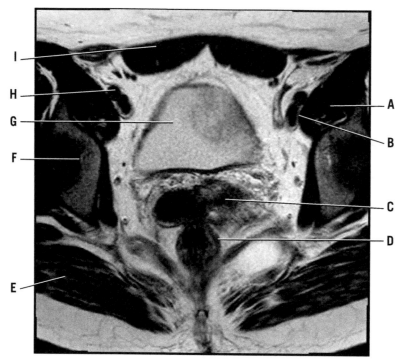

MR images provided courtesy of Roger Williams Medical Center.

A. _____

B. _____

C. _____

D. _____

E. _____

F. _____

G. _____

H. _____

I. _____

EXERCISE 7-31: LABELING

Label the following image from the list of terms provided in the Chapter 7 Word List in Appendix B.

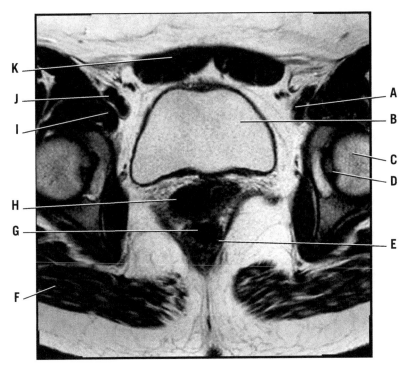

MR images provided courtesy of Roger Williams Medical Center.

A. _____

B. _____

C. _____

D. _____

E. _____

F. _____

G. _____

H. _____

I. _____

J. _____

K. _____

EXERCISE 7-32: LABELING

Label the following image from the list of terms provided in the Chapter 7 Word List in Appendix B.

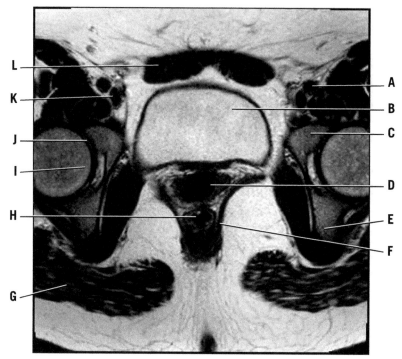

MR images provided courtesy of Roger Williams Medical Center.

A. _____

B. _____

C. _____

D. _____

E. _____

F. _____

G. _____

H. _____

I. _____

J. _____

K. _____

L. _____

EXERCISE 7-33: LABELING

Label the following image from the list of terms provided in the Chapter 7 Word List in Appendix B.

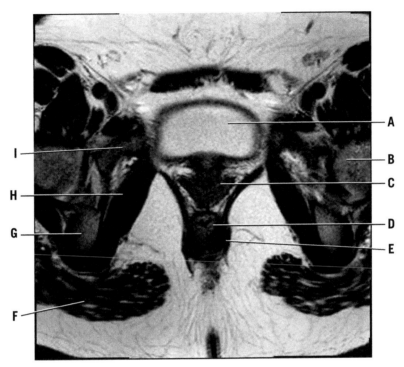

MR images provided courtesy of Roger Williams Medical Center.

A. _____

B. _____

C. _____

D. _____

E. _____

F. _____

G. _____

H. _____

I. _____

EXERCISE 7-34: LABELING

Label the following image from the list of terms provided in the Chapter 7 Word List in Appendix B.

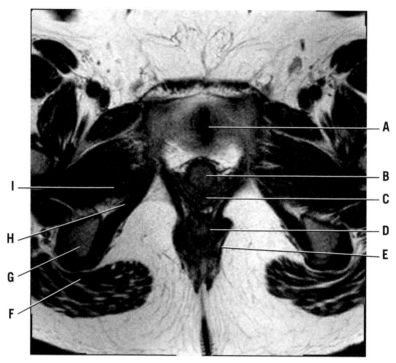

MR images provided courtesy of Roger Williams Medical Center.

A. _____

B. _____

C. _____

D. _____

E. _____

F. _____

G. _____

H. _____

I. _____

EXERCISE 7-35: LABELING

Label the following image from the list of terms provided in the Chapter 7 Word List in Appendix B.

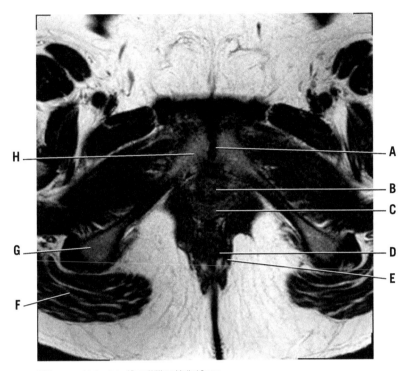

MR images provided courtesy of Roger Williams Medical Center.

A. _____

B. _____

C. _____

D. _____

E. _____

F. _____

G. _____

H. _____

EXERCISE 7-36: LABELING

Label the following image from the list of terms provided in the Chapter 7 Word List in Appendix B.

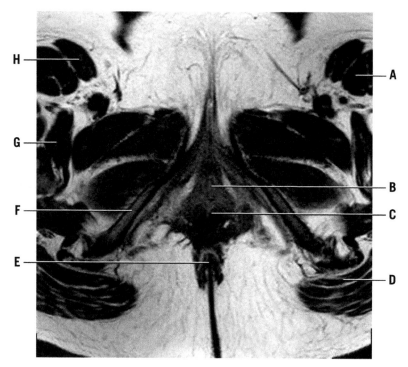

MR images provided courtesy of Roger Williams Medical Center.

A. _____

B. _____

C. _____

D. _____

E. _____

F. _____

G. _____

H. _____

EXERCISE 7-37: LABELING

Label the following image from the list of terms provided in the Chapter 7 Word List in Appendix B.

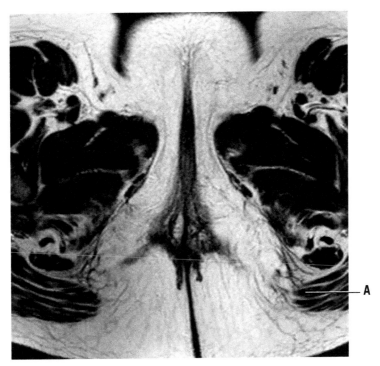

MR images provided courtesy of Roger Williams Medical Center.

A. _____

SAGITTAL IMAGES OF A FEMALE PELVIS

EXERCISE 7-38: LABELING

Label the following image from the list of terms provided in the Chapter 7 Word List in Appendix B.

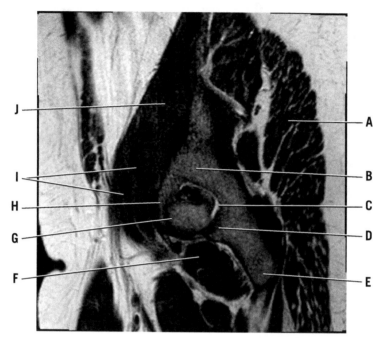

MR images provided courtesy of Roger Williams Medical Center.

A. _____

B. _____

C. _____

D. _____

E. _____

F. _____

G. _____

H. _____

I. _____

J. _____

EXERCISE 7-39: LABELING

Label the following image from the list of terms provided in the Chapter 7 Word List in Appendix B.

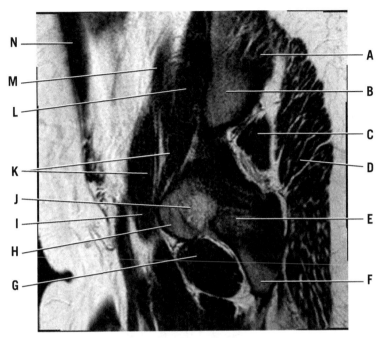

MR images provided courtesy of Roger Williams Medical Center.

A. _____

B. _____

C. _____

D. _____

E. _____

F. _____

G. _____

H. _____

I. _____

J. _____

K. _____

L. _____

M. _____

N. _____

EXERCISE 7-40: LABELING

Label the following image from the list of terms provided in the Chapter 7 Word List in Appendix B.

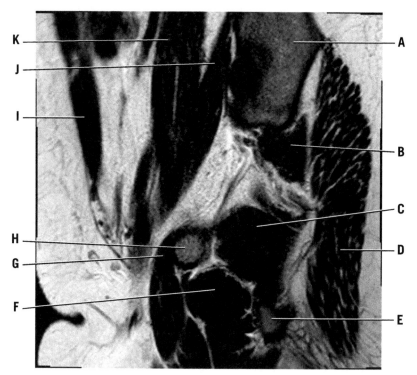

MR images provided courtesy of Roger Williams Medical Center.

A. _____

B. _____

C. _____

D. _____

E. _____

F. _____

G. _____

H. _____

I. _____

J. _____

K. _____

EXERCISE 7-41: LABELING

Label the following image from the list of terms provided in the Chapter 7 Word List in Appendix B.

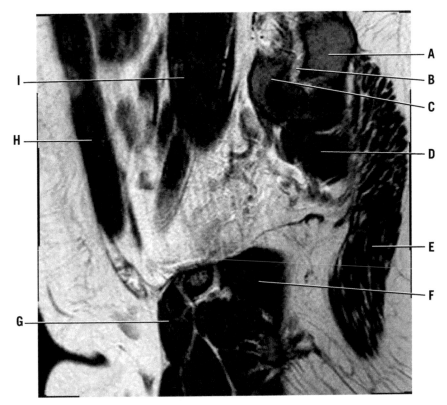

MR images provided courtesy of Roger Williams Medical Center.

A. _____

B. _____

C. _____

D. _____

E. _____

F. _____

G. _____

H. _____

I. _____

EXERCISE 7-42: LABELING

Label the following image from the list of terms provided in the Chapter 7 Word List in Appendix B.

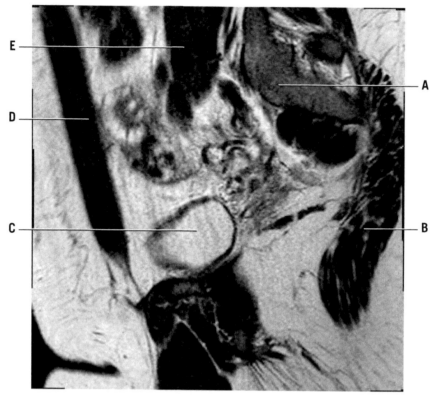

MR images provided courtesy of Roger Williams Medical Center.

A. _____

B. _____

C. _____

D. _____

E. _____

EXERCISE 7-43: LABELING

Label the following image from the list of terms provided in the Chapter 7 Word List in Appendix B.

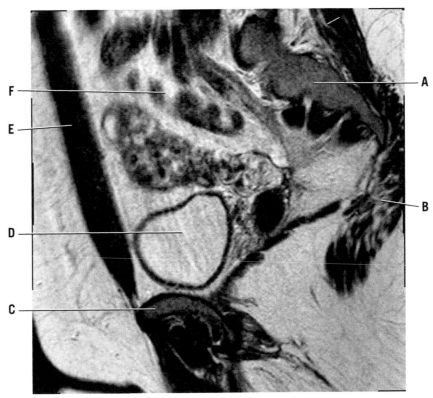

MR images provided courtesy of Roger Williams Medical Center.

A. _____

B. _____

C. _____

D. _____

E. _____

F. _____

EXERCISE 7-44: LABELING

Label the following image from the list of terms provided in the Chapter 7 Word List in Appendix B.

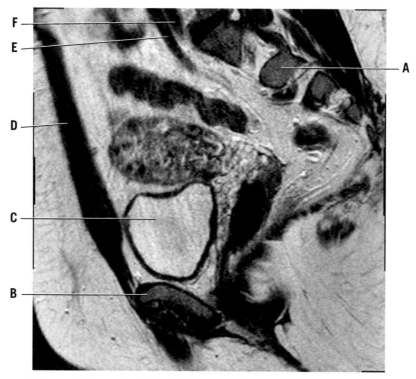

MR images provided courtesy of Roger Williams Medical Center.

A. _____

B. _____

C. _____

D. _____

E. _____

F. _____

EXERCISE 7-45: LABELING

Label the following image from the list of terms provided in the Chapter 7 Word List in Appendix B.

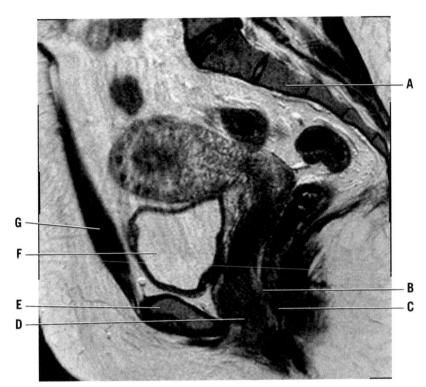

MR images provided courtesy of Roger Williams Medical Center.

A. _____

B. _____

C. _____

D. _____

E. _____

F. _____

G. _____

EXERCISE 7-46: LABELING

Label the following image from the list of terms provided in the Chapter 7 Word List in Appendix B.

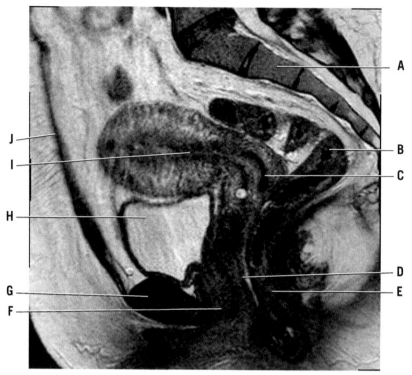

MR images provided courtesy of Roger Williams Medical Center.

A. _____

B. _____

C. _____

D. _____

E. _____

F. _____

G. _____

H. _____

I. _____

J. _____

EXERCISE 7-47: LABELING

Label the following image from the list of terms provided in the Chapter 7 Word List in Appendix B.

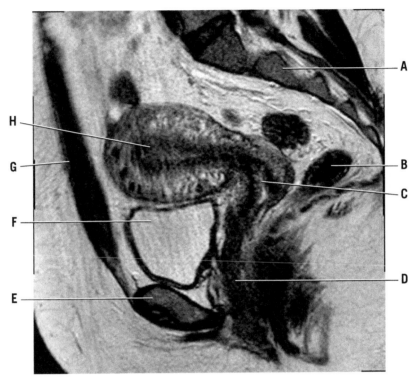

MR images provided courtesy of Roger Williams Medical Center.

A. _____

B. _____

C. _____

D. _____

E. _____

F. _____

G. _____

H. _____

EXERCISE 7-48: LABELING

Label the following image from the list of terms provided in the Chapter 7 Word List in Appendix B.

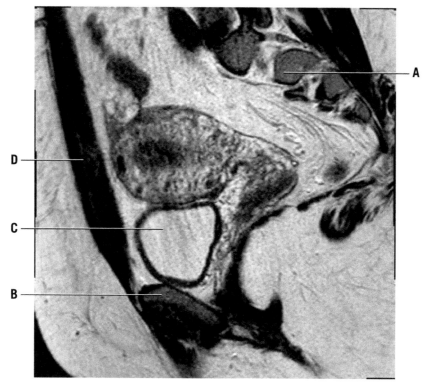

MR images provided courtesy of Roger Williams Medical Center.

A. _____

B. _____

C. _____

D. _____

EXERCISE 7-49: LABELING

Label the following image from the list of terms provided in the Chapter 7 Word List in Appendix B.

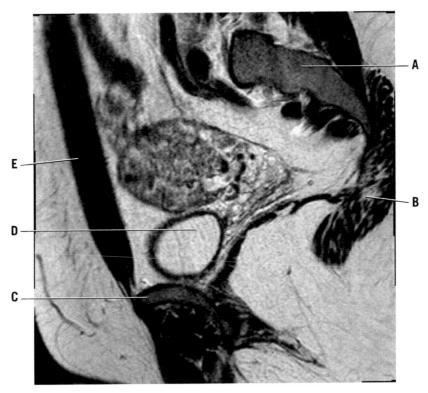

MR images provided courtesy of Roger Williams Medical Center.

A. _____

B. _____

C. _____

D. _____

E. _____

EXERCISE 7-50: LABELING

Label the following image from the list of terms provided in the Chapter 7 Word List in Appendix B.

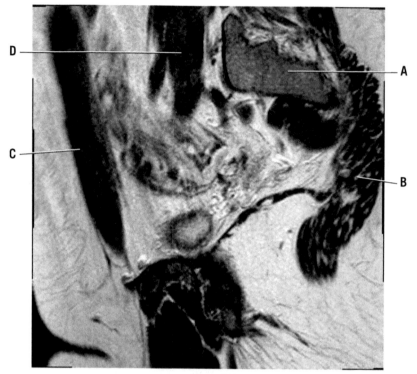

MR images provided courtesy of Roger Williams Medical Center.

A. _____

B. _____

C. _____

D. _____

EXERCISE 7-51: LABELING

Label the following image from the list of terms provided in the Chapter 7 Word List in Appendix B.

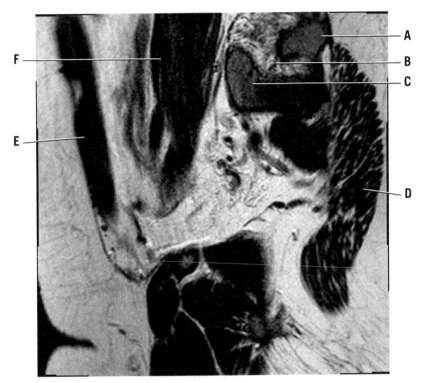

MR images provided courtesy of Roger Williams Medical Center.

A. _____

B. _____

C. _____

D. _____

E. _____

F. _____

EXERCISE 7-52: LABELING

Label the following image from the list of terms provided in the Chapter 7 Word List in Appendix B.

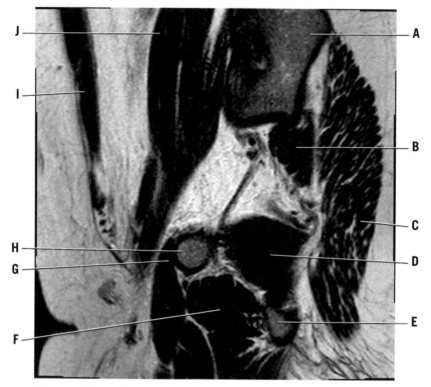

MR images provided courtesy of Roger Williams Medical Center.

A. _____

B. _____

C. _____

D. _____

E. _____

F. _____

G. _____

H. _____

I. _____

J. _____

EXERCISE 7-53: LABELING

Label the following image from the list of terms provided in the **Chapter 7 Word List** in **Appendix B.**

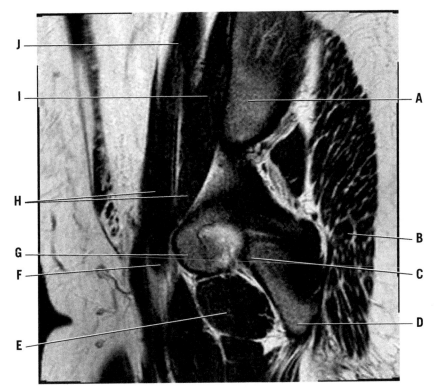

MR images provided courtesy of Roger Williams Medical Center.

A. _____

B. _____

C. _____

D. _____

E. _____

F. _____

G. _____

H. _____

I. _____

J. _____

EXERCISE 7-54: LABELING

Label the following image from the list of terms provided in the Chapter 7 Word List in Appendix B.

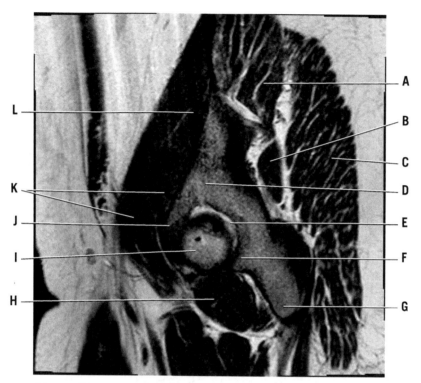

MR images provided courtesy of Roger Williams Medical Center.

A. _____

B. _____

C. _____

D. _____

E. _____

F. _____

G. _____

H. _____

I. _____

J. _____

K. _____

L. _____

Vertebral Column

OUTLINE

EXERCISE 8-1: LABELING

Label the following illustration from the list of terms provided.

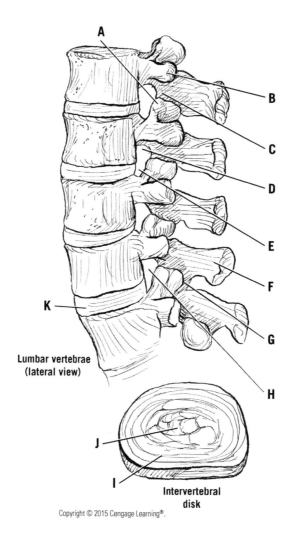

Lumbar vertebrae
(lateral view)

Intervertebral
disk

annulus fibrosus

apophyseal joint

inferior articular process

inferior vertebral notch

intervertebral disc

intervertebral foramen

nucleus pulposus

spinous process

superior articular process

superior vertebral notch

transverse process

A. _____

B. _____

C. _____

D. _____

E. _____

F. _____

G. _____

H. _____

I. _____

J. _____

K. _____

EXERCISE 8-2: MATCHING

Match the following terms with the correct definition.

____ 1. annulus fibrosus

____ 2. atlas

____ 3. cauda equina

____ 4. kyphosis

____ 5. PLL

a. an exaggerated posterior convex curvature of the spinal column in the thoracic region

b. ring-shaped outer edge of an intervertebral disk

c. a ligament running along the posterior aspect of the bodies of the vertebrae

d. the first cervical vertebra

e. the hairlike nerve roots extending from the tapered end of the spinal cord

EXERCISE 8-3: IDENTIFICATION

Identify the seven processes associated with the vertebral arch.

1. _____

2. _____

3. _____

4. _____

5. _____

6. _____

7. _____

EXERCISE 8-4: COMPLETION

Complete the following blanks by selecting the correct terms from the list provided.

cauda equina   coccyx   foramen magnum   pia mater
cervical   conus medullaris   lumbar   spinal nerves
coccygeal   filium terminale   medulla oblongata   vertebral canal

The spinal cord extends below the _____ as a continuation of the

_____. It is thicker in the _____ and _____

regions and passes through the _____. The tapered end of the spinal cord, the

_____, has hairlike nerve extensions, the _____. Anchoring

the spinal cord to the _____ is the _____, an extension of the

_____. Attached to the spinal cord are 31 pairs of _____, one

for each vertebra, with the exception of the _____ region, which has eight and the

_____ region, which has one.

EXERCISE 8-5: MATCHING

Match the following ligaments associated with the vertebral column with the correct definitions.

____ 1. anterior longitudinal

____ 2. ligamentum flava

____ 3. ligamentum nuchae

____ 4. posterior longitudinal ligament

____ 5. supraspinous ligament

a. a ligament running along the medial aspect of the laminae of the vertebrae

b. a ligament running along the anterior aspect of the bodies of the vertebrae

c. a ligament running along the tips of the spinous processes of the vertebrae from C7 to the occipital bone

d. a ligament running along the tips of the spinous processes of the vertebrae from C7 to the sacrum

e. a ligament running along the posterior aspect of the bodies of the vertebrae

EXERCISE 8-6: LABELING

Label the following illustration from the list of terms provided.

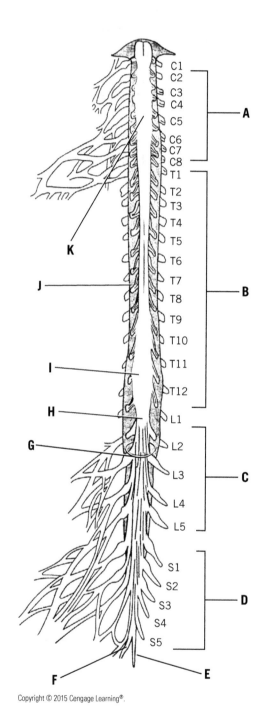

cauda equina
cervical enlargement
cervical spinal nerves
coccygeal nerve
conus medullaris
dura mater
filium terminale
lumbar enlargement
lumbar spinal nerves
sacral spinal nerves
thoracic spinal nerves

A. _____

B. _____

C. _____

D. _____

E. _____

F. _____

G. _____

H. _____

I. _____

J. _____

K. _____

CT AXIAL IMAGES

EXERCISE 8-7: LABELING

Label the following image from the list of terms provided in the **Chapter 8 Word List** in **Appendix B.**

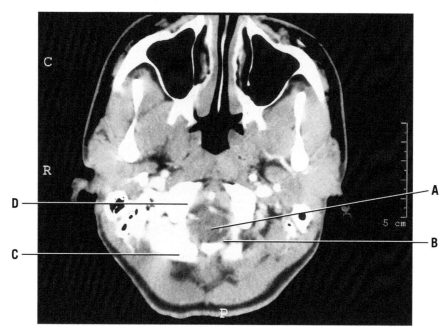

CT Images provided courtesy of Roger Williams Medical Center.

A. _____

B. _____

C. _____

D. _____

EXERCISE 8-8: LABELING

Label the following image from the list of terms provided in the Chapter 8 Word List in Appendix B.

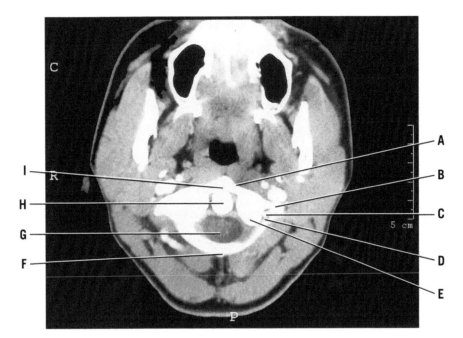

CT Images provided courtesy of Roger Williams Medical Center.

A. _____

B. _____

C. _____

D. _____

E. _____

F. _____

G. _____

H. _____

I. _____

EXERCISE 8-9: LABELING

Label the following image from the list of terms provided in the **Chapter 8 Word List** in **Appendix B.**

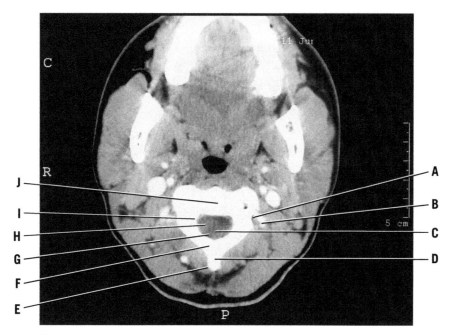

CT Images provided courtesy of Roger Williams Medical Center.

A. _____

B. _____

C. _____

D. _____

E. _____

F. _____

G. _____

H. _____

I. _____

J. _____

EXERCISE 8-10: LABELING

Label the following image from the list of terms provided in the Chapter 8 Word List in Appendix B.

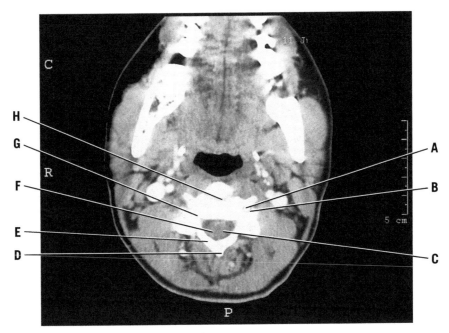

CT Images provided courtesy of Roger Williams Medical Center.

A. _____

B. _____

C. _____

D. _____

E. _____

F. _____

G. _____

H. _____

EXERCISE 8-11: LABELING

Label the following image from the list of terms provided in the Chapter 8 Word List in Appendix B.

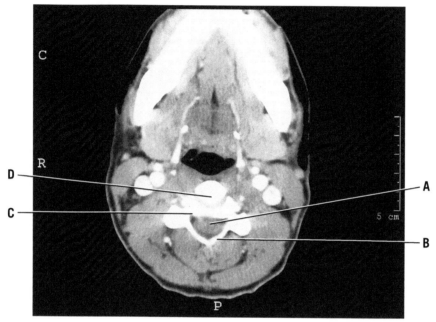

CT Images provided courtesy of Roger Williams Medical Center.

A. _____

B. _____

C. _____

D. _____

EXERCISE 8-12: LABELING

Label the following image from the list of terms provided in the Chapter 8 Word List in Appendix B.

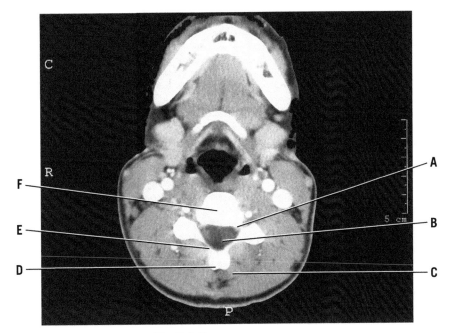

CT Images provided courtesy of Roger Williams Medical Center.

A. _____

B. _____

C. _____

D. _____

E. _____

F. _____

EXERCISE 8-13: LABELING

Label the following image from the list of terms provided in the Chapter 8 Word List in Appendix B.

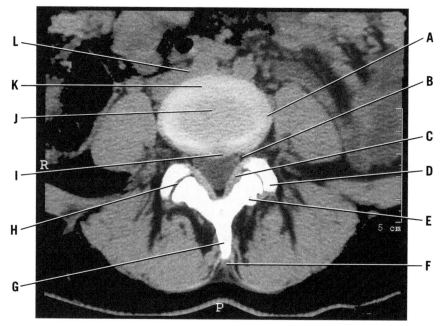

CT Images provided courtesy of Roger Williams Medical Center.

A. _____

B. _____

C. _____

D. _____

E. _____

F. _____

G. _____

H. _____

I. _____

J. _____

K. _____

L. _____

EXERCISE 8-14: LABELING

Label the following image from the list of terms provided in the **Chapter 8 Word List** in Appendix B.

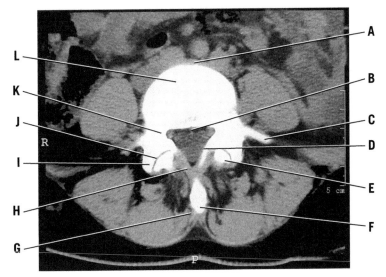

CT Images provided courtesy of Roger Williams Medical Center.

A. _____

B. _____

C. _____

D. _____

E. _____

F. _____

G. _____

H. _____

I. _____

J. _____

K. _____

L. _____

EXERCISE 8-15: LABELING

Label the following image from the list of terms provided in the Chapter 8 Word List in Appendix B.

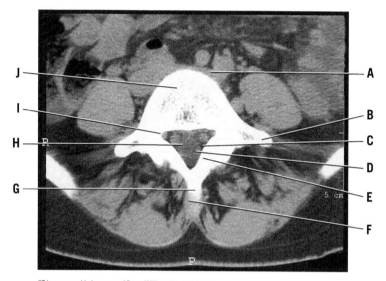

CT Images provided courtesy of Roger Williams Medical Center.

A. _____

B. _____

C. _____

D. _____

E. _____

F. _____

G. _____

H. _____

I. _____

J. _____

EXERCISE 8-16: LABELING

Label the following image from the list of terms provided in the Chapter 8 Word List in Appendix B.

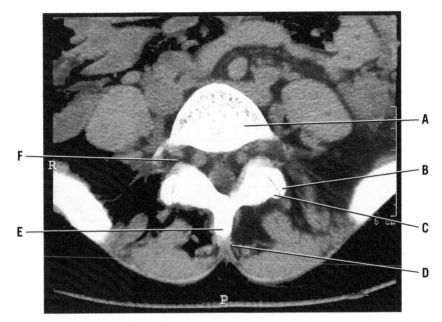

CT Images provided courtesy of Roger Williams Medical Center.

A. _____

B. _____

C. _____

D. _____

E. _____

F. _____

EXERCISE 8-17: LABELING

Label the following image from the list of terms provided in the Chapter 8 Word List in Appendix B.

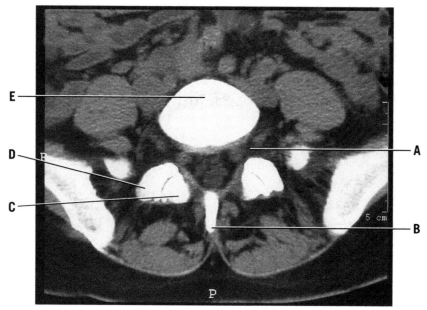

CT Images provided courtesy of Roger Williams Medical Center.

A. _____

B. _____

C. _____

D. _____

E. _____

EXERCISE 8-18: LABELING

Label the following image from the list of terms provided in the **Chapter 8 Word List** in **Appendix B.**

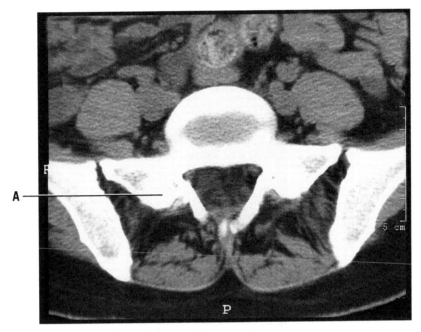

CT Images provided courtesy of Roger Williams Medical Center.

A. _____

MR IMAGES

SAGITTAL IMAGES

EXERCISE 8-19: LABELING

Label the following image from the list of terms provided in the Chapter 8 Word List in Appendix B.

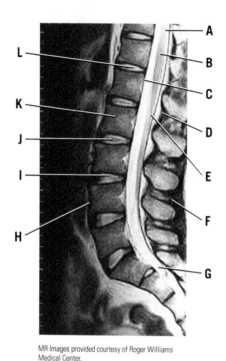

MR Images provided courtesy of Roger Williams Medical Center.

A. _____ G. _____

B. _____ H. _____

C. _____ I. _____

D. _____ J. _____

E. _____ K. _____

F. _____ L. _____

EXERCISE 8-20: LABELING

Label the following image from the list of terms provided in the Chapter 8 Word List in Appendix B.

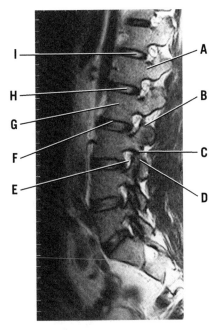

MR Images provided courtesy of Roger Williams Medical Center.

A. _____

B. _____

C. _____

D. _____

E. _____

F. _____

G. _____

H. _____

I. _____

AXIAL IMAGES

EXERCISE 8-21: LABELING

Label the following image from the list of terms provided in the Chapter 8 Word List in Appendix B.

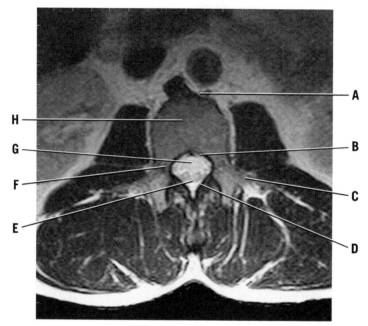

MR Images provided courtesy of Roger Williams Medical Center.

A. _____

B. _____

C. _____

D. _____

E. _____

F. _____

G. _____

H. _____

EXERCISE 8-22: LABELING

Label the following image from the list of terms provided in the Chapter 8 Word List in Appendix B.

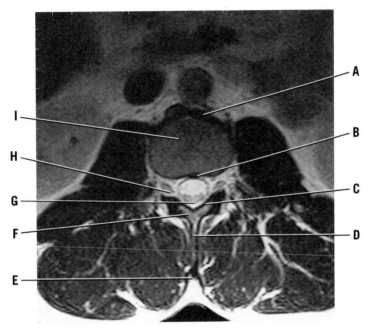

MR Images provided courtesy of Roger Williams Medical Center.

A. _____

B. _____

C. _____

D. _____

E. _____

F. _____

G. _____

H. _____

I. _____

EXERCISE 8-23: LABELING

Label the following image from the list of terms provided in the Chapter 8 Word List in Appendix B.

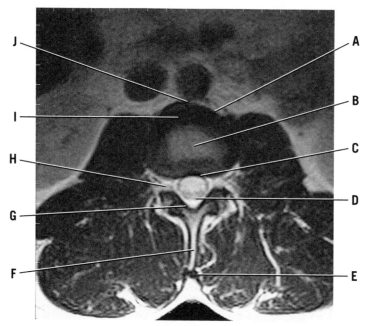

MR Images provided courtesy of Roger Williams Medical Center.

A. _____

B. _____

C. _____

D. _____

E. _____

F. _____

G. _____

H. _____

I. _____

J. _____

EXERCISE 8-24: LABELING

Label the following image from the list of terms provided in the Chapter 8 Word List in Appendix B.

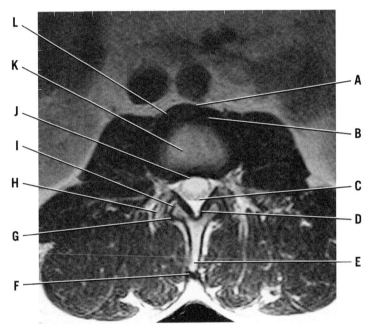

MR Images provided courtesy of Roger Williams Medical Center.

A. _____

B. _____

C. _____

D. _____

E. _____

F. _____

G. _____

H. _____

I. _____

J. _____

K. _____

L. _____

EXERCISE 8-25: LABELING

Label the following image from the list of terms provided in the Chapter 8 Word List in Appendix B.

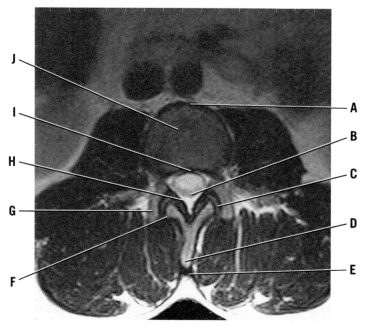

MR Images provided courtesy of Roger Williams Medical Center.

A. _____

B. _____

C. _____

D. _____

E. _____

F. _____

G. _____

H. _____

I. _____

J. _____

EXERCISE 8-26: LABELING

Label the following image from the list of terms provided in the Chapter 8 Word List in Appendix B.

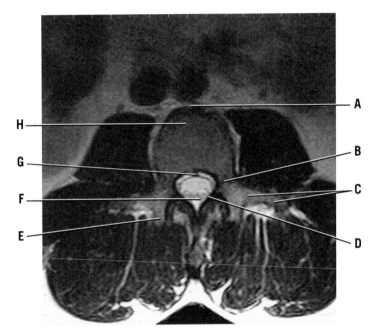

MR Images provided courtesy of Roger Williams Medical Center.

A. _____

B. _____

C. _____

D. _____

E. _____

F. _____

G. _____

H. _____

Upper Extremity

OUTLINE

EXERCISE 9-1: MATCHING

Match the following terms with the correct definitions.

—— 1. appendicular skeleton

—— 2. axial skeleton

—— 3. diarthrodial joint

—— 4. synovial joint

a. a freely movable joint with an enclosed joint cavity

b. the upper and lower extremities and pelvic and shoulder girdles

c. a cartilaginous or slightly movable joint

d. skull, three auditory ossicles, hyoid bone, sternum, ribs, and bones of the vertebral column

EXERCISE 9-2: TERM IDENTIFICATION

Identify the following definitions as describing: (A) ball-and-socket joint, (B) condyloid joint, (C) hinge joint, or (D) pivot joint.

—— 1. a type of synovial joint allowing for rotation only where an extension of one bone fits into a bony/ligamentous ring of another

—— 2. a type of synovial joint in which the articulating bones can move in only one plane, anteriorly and posteriorly, with the bones moving in opposite directions

—— 3. a type of synovial joint where a portion of one bone fits into an elliptical cavity of another, permitting movement in two axes (for example, up and down or side to side), but not axial rotation

—— 4. a type of synovial joint in which a rounded head of one bone fits into a cup-shaped cavity of another, permitting virtually unlimited movement

EXERCISE 9-3: IDENTIFICATION

List the bones in the axial skeleton.

1. _____

2. _____

3. _____

4. _____

5. _____

6. _____

EXERCISE 9-4: IDENTIFICATION

List the bones in the appendicular skeleton.

1. _____

2. _____

3. _____

4. _____

EXERCISE 9-5: MATCHING

Match the following landmarks with the appropriate bones.

____ 1. conoid tubercle

____ 2. coracoid process

____ 3. coronoid process

____ 4. trochlea

____ 5. ulna notch

a. clavicle

b. humerus

c. radius

d. scapula

e. ulna

EXERCISE 9-6: IDENTIFICATION

Indicate whether the following landmarks of the upper extremity are located (A) anteriorly or (B) posteriorly on the associated bones.

____ 1. capitulum

____ 2. coracoid process

____ 3. coronoid fossa

____ 4. coronoid process

____ 5. infraspinous fossa

____ 6. intertubercular groove

____ 7. olecranon

____ 8. olecranon fossa

____ 9. radial fossa

____ 10. spinous process

____ 11. subscapular fossa

____ 12. supraspinous fossa

____ 13. trochlea

EXERCISE 9-7: IDENTIFICATION

Identify the following muscles as (A) muscles that move the humerus, (B) muscles that move the radius and ulna, or (C) muscles that move the hand.

____ 1. anconeus

____ 2. biceps brachii

____ 3. brachialis

____ 4. coracobrachialis

____ 5. deltoid

____ 6. extensor

____ 7. flexor

____ 8. pronator quadratus

____ 9. teres major

____ 10. teres minor

EXERCISE 9-8: IDENTIFICATION

List the muscles involved in the rotator cuff.

1. _____

2. _____

3. _____

4. _____

EXERCISE 9-9: IDENTIFICATION

Classify the following joints as being (A) amphiarthrodial, (B) diarthrodial, or (C) synarthrodial.

____ 1. elbow joint

____ 2. shoulder joint

____ 3. wrist joint

EXERCISE 9-10: IDENTIFICATION

Indicate whether the ligaments listed are associated with the (A) elbow joint, (B) shoulder joint, or (C) wrist joint.

_____ 1. annular

_____ 2. coracohumeral

_____ 3. dorsal carpal

_____ 4. flexor retinaculum manus

_____ 5. glenohumeral

_____ 6. palmar carpal

_____ 7. transverse humeral

EXERCISE 9-11: SORTING

Which one of the following does not belong in this list?

1. extensor tendons

2. flexor retinaculum manus

3. flexor tendons

4. median nerve

EXERCISE 9-12: MATCHING

Match the following articulations with the type of synovial joint.

_____ 1. humerus, radius, and ulna

_____ 2. proximal radius and ulna

_____ 3. radius, scaphoid, lunate, and triquetrum

_____ 4. shoulder joint

a. ball-and-socket

b. condyloid

c. hinge

d. pivot

EXERCISE 9-13: LABELING

Label the following illustration from the list of terms provided.

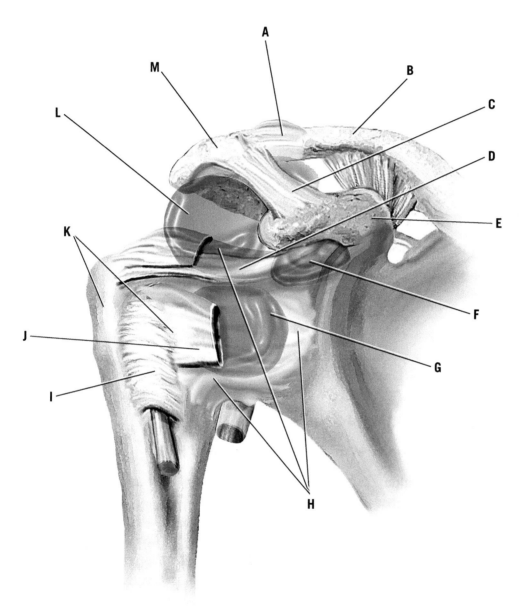

acromioclavicular ligaments

acromion

clavicle

coracoacromial ligament

coracohumeral ligament

coracoid process

glenohumeral ligament

greater and lesser tubercles of the humerus

subacromial/subdeltoid bursa

subcoracoid bursa

subscapularis bursa

subscapularis tendon (cut)

transverse humeral ligament

A. _____

B. _____

C. _____

D. _____

E. _____

F. _____

G. _____

H. _____

I. _____

J. _____

K. _____

L. _____

M. _____

EXERCISE 9-14: LABELING

Label the following illustration from the list of terms provided.

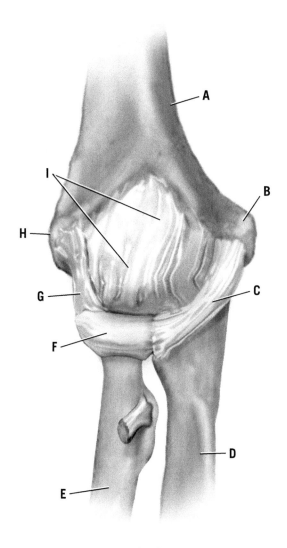

**Anterior view
of right elbow**

annular ligament of the radius

humerus

joint capsule

lateral epicondyle

medial epicondyle

radial collateral ligament

radius

ulna

ulnar collateral ligament

A. _____

B. _____

C. _____

D. _____

E. _____

F. _____

G. _____

H. _____

I. _____

EXERCISE 9-15: LABELING

Label the following illustration from the list of terms provided.

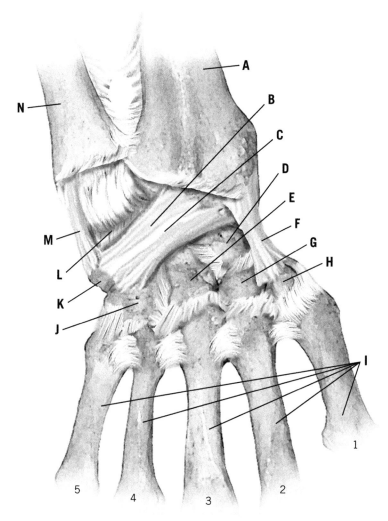

capitate bone
dorsal radiocarpal ligament
dorsal ulnocarpal ligament
hamate bone
lunate bone
metacarpal bones
radial collateral ligament
radius
scaphoid bone
trapezium
trapezoid bone
triquetrum bone
ulna
ulnar collateral ligament

A. _____

B. _____

C. _____

D. _____

E. _____

F. _____

G. _____

H. _____

I. _____

J. _____

K. _____

L. _____

M. _____

N. _____

EXERCISE 9-16: TERM IDENTIFICATION

Provide a synonym for the following terms.

1. brachioradialis muscle _____

2. diarthrodial joint _____

3. dorsal carpal ligament _____

4. intertubercular groove _____

5. palmar carpal ligament _____

6. radial collateral ligament _____

7. shoulder joint _____

8. ulnar collateral ligament _____

CT AXIAL IMAGES OF THE SHOULDER

EXERCISE 9-17: LABELING

Label the following image from the list of terms provided in the Chapter 9 Word List in Appendix B.

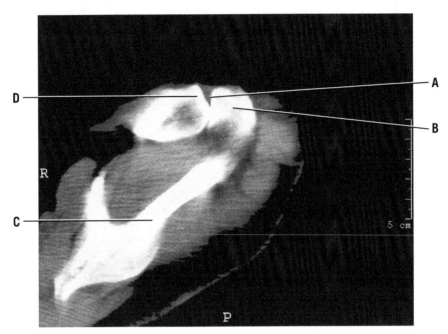

CT Images provided by Our Lady of Fatima Hospital, North Providence, Rhode Island and Roger Williams Medical Center.

A. _____

B. _____

C. _____

D. _____

EXERCISE 9-18: LABELING

Label the following image from the list of terms provided in the Chapter 9 Word List in Appendix B.

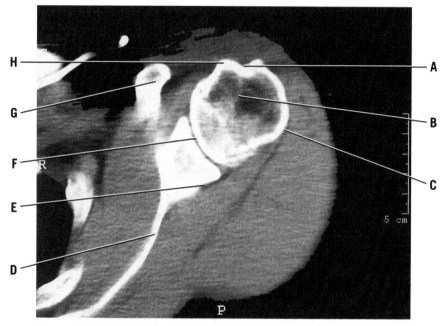

CT Images provided by Our Lady of Fatima Hospital, North Providence, Rhode Island and Roger Williams Medical Center.

A. _____

B. _____

C. _____

D. _____

E. _____

F. _____

G. _____

H. _____

EXERCISE 9-19: LABELING

Label the following image from the list of terms provided in the Chapter 9 Word List in Appendix B.

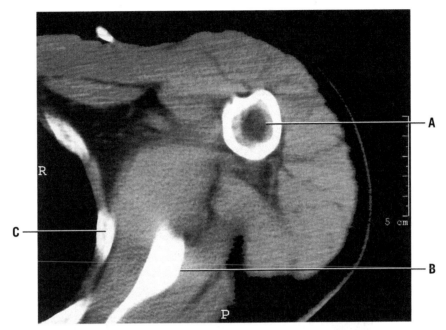

CT Images provided by Our Lady of Fatima Hospital, North Providence, Rhode Island and Roger Williams Medical Center.

A. _____

B. _____

C. _____

MR IMAGES OF THE SHOULDER

AXIAL IMAGE

EXERCISE 9-20: LABELING

Label the following image from the list of terms provided in the Chapter 9 Word List in Appendix B.

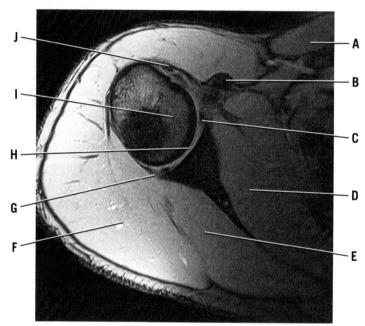

MR Images provided by Roger Williams Medical Center.

A. _____

B. _____

C. _____

D. _____

E. _____

F. _____

G. _____

H. _____

I. _____

J. _____

CORONAL IMAGE

EXERCISE 9-21: LABELING

Label the following image from the list of terms provided in the Chapter 9 Word List in Appendix B.

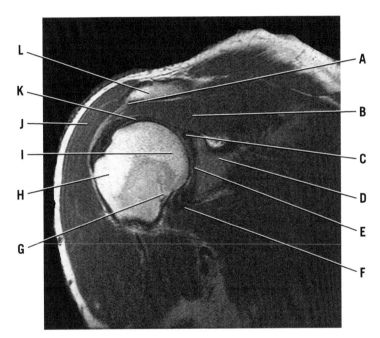

MR Images provided by Roger Williams Medical Center.

A. _____

B. _____

C. _____

D. _____

E. _____

F. _____

G. _____

H. _____

I. _____

J. _____

K. _____

L. _____

SAGITTAL IMAGE

EXERCISE 9-22: LABELING

Label the following image from the list of terms provided in the Chapter 9 Word List in Appendix B.

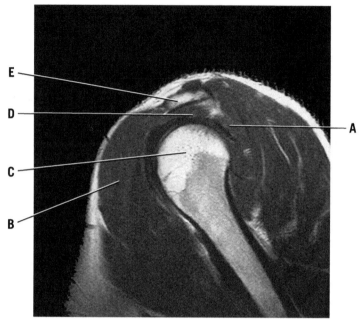

MR Images provided by Roger Williams Medical Center.

A. _____

B. _____

C. _____

D. _____

E. _____

CT AXIAL IMAGES OF THE ELBOW

EXERCISE 9-23: LABELING

Label the following image from the list of terms provided in the Chapter 9 Word List in Appendix B.

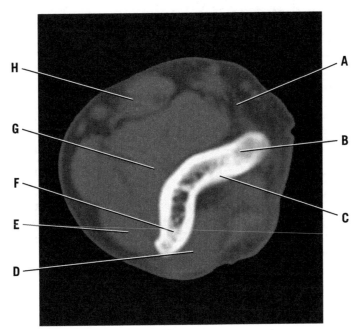

CT Images provided by Our Lady of Fatima Hospital, North Providence, Rhode Island and Roger Williams Medical Center.

A. _____

B. _____

C. _____

D. _____

E. _____

F. _____

G. _____

H. _____

EXERCISE 9-24: LABELING

Label the following image from the list of terms provided in the Chapter 9 Word List in Appendix B.

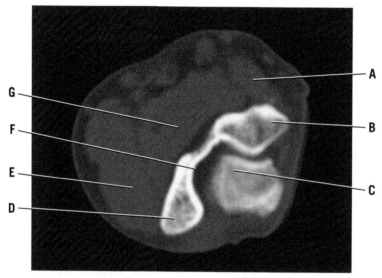

CT Images provided by Our Lady of Fatima Hospital, North Providence, Rhode Island and Roger Williams Medical Center.

A. _____

B. _____

C. _____

D. _____

E. _____

F. _____

G. _____

EXERCISE 9-25: LABELING

Label the following image from the list of terms provided in the Chapter 9 Word List in Appendix B.

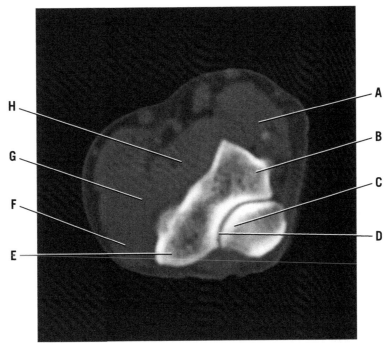

CT Images provided by Our Lady of Fatima Hospital, North Providence, Rhode Island and Roger Williams Medical Center.

A. _____

B. _____

C. _____

D. _____

E. _____

F. _____

G. _____

H. _____

EXERCISE 9-26: LABELING

Label the following image from the list of terms provided in the **Chapter 9 Word List** in Appendix B.

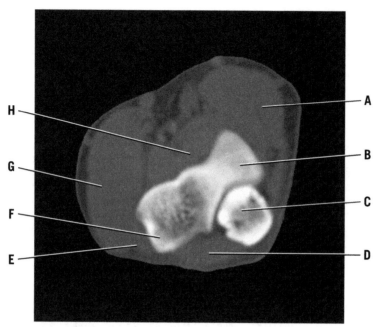

CT Images provided by Our Lady of Fatima Hospital, North Providence, Rhode Island and Roger Williams Medical Center.

A. _____

B. _____

C. _____

D. _____

E. _____

F. _____

G. _____

H. _____

EXERCISE 9-27: LABELING

Label the following image from the list of terms provided in the Chapter 9 Word List in Appendix B.

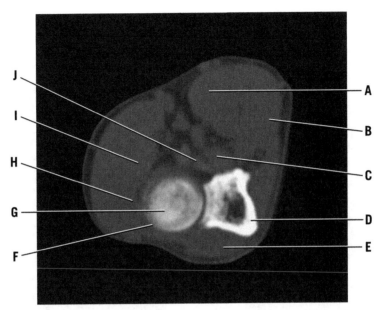

CT Images provided by Our Lady of Fatima Hospital, North Providence, Rhode Island and Roger Williams Medical Center.

A. _____

B. _____

C. _____

D. _____

E. _____

F. _____

G. _____

H. _____

I. _____

J. _____

MR IMAGES OF THE ELBOW

EXERCISE 9-28: LABELING

Label the following image from the list of terms provided in the Chapter 9 Word List in Appendix B.

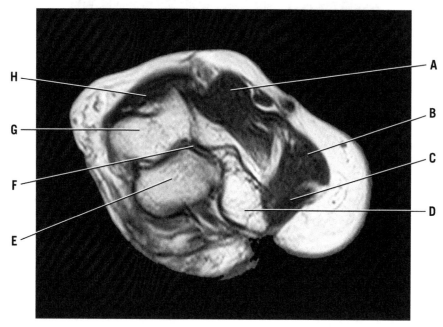

MR Images provided by Roger Williams Medical Center.

A. _____

B. _____

C. _____

D. _____

E. _____

F. _____

G. _____

H. _____

CORONAL IMAGES

AXIAL IMAGE

EXERCISE 9-29: LABELING

Label the following image from the list of terms provided in the Chapter 9 Word List in Appendix B.

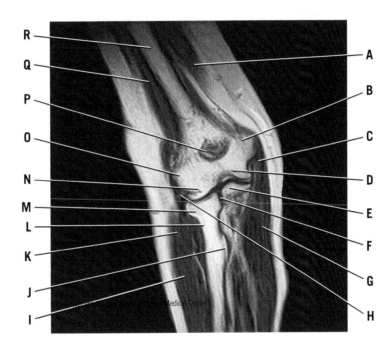

A. _____

B. _____

C. _____

D. _____

E. _____

F. _____

G. _____

H. _____

I. _____

J. _____

K. _____

L. _____

M. _____

N. _____

O. _____

P. _____

Q. _____

R. _____

EXERCISE 9-30: LABELING

Label the following image from the list of terms provided in the Chapter 9 Word List in Appendix B.

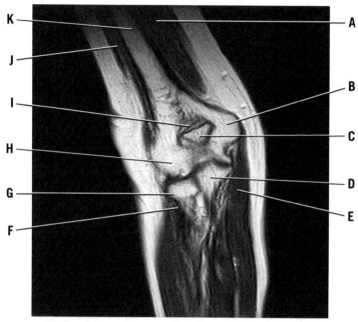

MR Images provided by Roger Williams Medical Center.

A. _____

B. _____

C. _____

D. _____

E. _____

F. _____

G. _____

H. _____

I. _____

J. _____

K. _____

CT IMAGES OF THE WRIST

EXERCISE 9-31: LABELING

Label the following image from the list of terms provided in the Chapter 9 Word List in Appendix B.

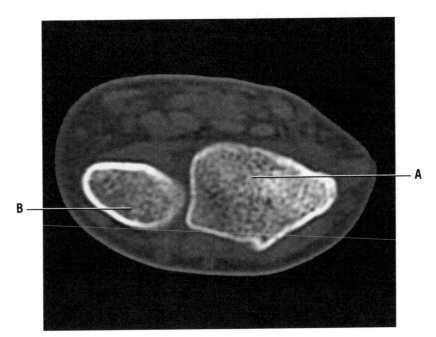

CT Images provided by Our Lady of Fatima Hospital, North Providence, Rhode Island and Roger Williams Medical Center.

A. _____

B. _____

EXERCISE 9-32: LABELING

Label the following image from the list of terms provided in the Chapter 9 Word List in Appendix B.

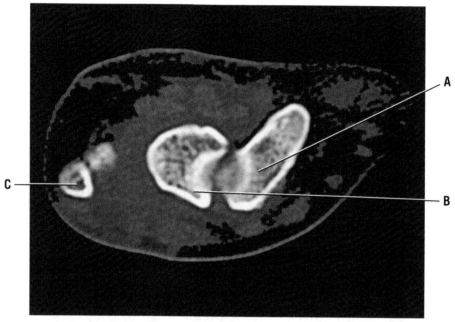

CT Images provided by Our Lady of Fatima Hospital, North Providence, Rhode Island and Roger Williams Medical Center.

A. _____

B. _____

C. _____

EXERCISE 9-33: LABELING

Label the following image from the list of terms provided in the Chapter 9 Word List in Appendix B.

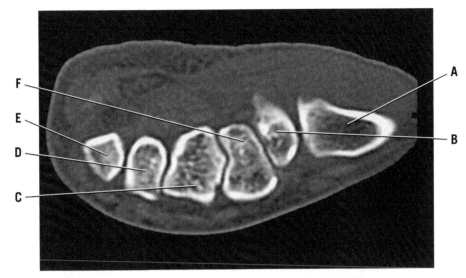

CT Images provided by Our Lady of Fatima Hospital, North Providence, Rhode Island and Roger Williams Medical Center.

A. _____

B. _____

C. _____

D. _____

E. _____

F. _____

MR IMAGES OF THE WRIST

AXIAL IMAGES

EXERCISE 9-34: LABELING

Label the following image from the list of terms provided in the **Chapter 9 Word List in Appendix B.**

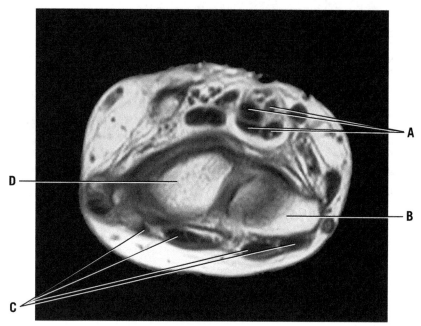

MR Images provided by Roger Williams Medical Center.

A. _____

B. _____

C. _____

D. _____

EXERCISE 9-35: LABELING

Label the following image from the list of terms provided in the Chapter 9 Word List in Appendix B.

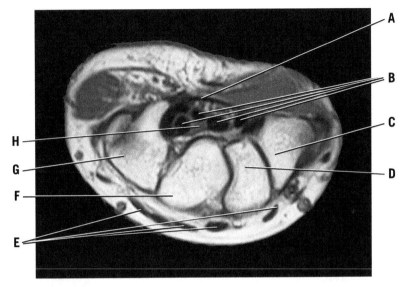

MR Images provided by Roger Williams Medical Center.

A. _____

B. _____

C. _____

D. _____

E. _____

F. _____

G. _____

H. _____

CORONAL IMAGES

EXERCISE 9-36: LABELING

Label the following image from the list of terms provided in the Chapter 9 Word List in Appendix B.

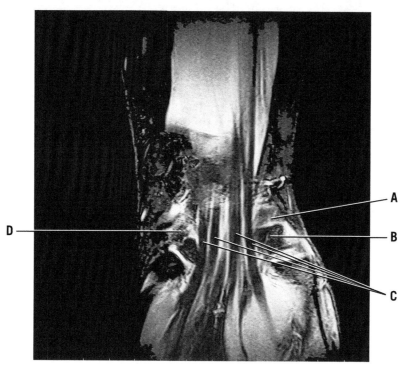

MR Images provided by Roger Williams Medical Center.

A. _____

B. _____

C. _____

D. _____

EXERCISE 9-37: LABELING

Label the following image from the list of terms provided in the Chapter 9 Word List in Appendix B.

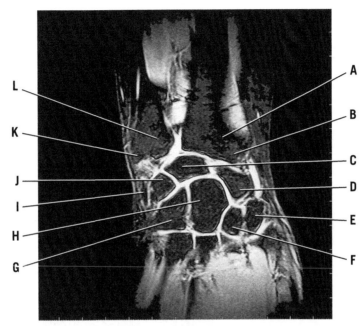

MR Images provided by Roger Williams Medical Center.

A. _____

B. _____

C. _____

D. _____

E. _____

F. _____

G. _____

H. _____

I. _____

J. _____

K. _____

L. _____

SAGITTAL IMAGES

EXERCISE 9-38: LABELING

Label the following image from the list of terms provided in the Chapter 9 Word List in Appendix B.

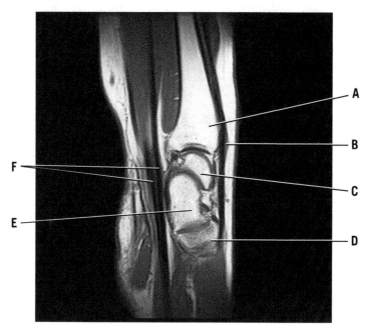

MR Images provided by Roger Williams Medical Center.

A. _____

B. _____

C. _____

D. _____

E. _____

F. _____

EXERCISE 9-39: LABELING

Label the following image from the list of terms provided in the Chapter 9 Word List in Appendix B.

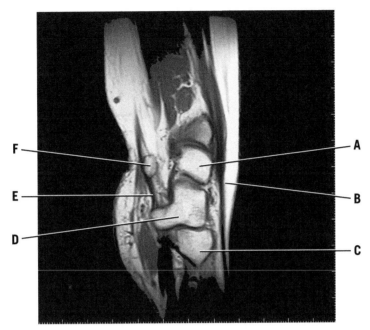

MR Images provided by Roger Williams Medical Center.

A. _____

B. _____

C. _____

D. _____

E. _____

F. _____

Lower Extremity

EXERCISE 10-1: IDENTIFICATION

Identify the bones of the lower extremity.

A. _____

B. _____

C. _____

D. _____

E. _____

F. _____

G. _____

EXERCISE 10-2: IDENTIFICATION

Indicate which bone the following landmarks are associated with: (A) femur, (B) tibia, or (C) fibula.

____ 1. fovea capitis

____ 2. intercondylar fossa

____ 3. intercondyloid eminence

____ 4. lateral malleolus

____ 5. linea aspera

____ 6. medial malleolus

____ 7. patellar surface

____ 8. styloid process

EXERCISE 10-3: IDENTIFICATION

Identify the seven tarsal bones.

A. _____

B. _____

C. _____

D. _____

E. _____

F. _____

G. _____

EXERCISE 10-4: TERM IDENTIFICATION

Provide a synonym for the following terms.

1. ankle joint   _____

2. big toe   _____

3. calcaneus   _____

4. femur   _____

5. first cuneiform   _____

6. talus   _____

EXERCISE 10-5: IDENTIFICATION

Identify the two muscle tendons forming the Achilles tendon.

1. _____

2. _____

EXERCISE 10-6: MATCHING

Match the following terms with the correct definitions.

___ 1. ankle joint   a. amphiarthrosis

___ 2. hip joint   b. diarthrosis

___ 3. knee joint   c. synarthrosis

EXERCISE 10-7: MATCHING

Match the following terms with the correct definitions. Some definitions may be used more than once.

___ 1. ankle joint   a. ball-and-socket

___ 2. hip joint   b. gliding

___ 3. knee joint   c. condyloid

                            d. hinge

EXERCISE 10-8: IDENTIFICATION

Indicate with which joint the following ligaments are associated: (A) ankle joint, (B) hip joint, or (C) knee joint.

_____ 1. anterior/posterior cruciate

_____ 2. arcuate popliteal

_____ 3. capsular

_____ 4. cotyloid

_____ 5. deltoid

_____ 6. interosseous

_____ 7. lateral collateral

_____ 8. ligamentum teres femoris

_____ 9. spring

EXERCISE 10-9: IDENTIFICATION

Indicate whether the following muscles that move the femur are in the (A) anterior group, (B) posterior group, (C) medial group, or (D) lateral group.

_____ 1. adductors

_____ 2. gluteal maximus

_____ 3. hamstring

_____ 4. inferior/superior gemellus

_____ 5. obturator externus/internus

_____ 6. pectineus

_____ 7. rectus femoris

_____ 8. sartorius

_____ 9. tensor

EXERCISE 10-10: IDENTIFICATION

For the following muscles that move the femur, indicate which action they perform: (A) flex the thigh at the hip joint, (B) laterally rotate, (C) adduct the thigh at the hip joint, or (D) abduct the thigh.

_____ 1. gluteal minimus

_____ 2. gracilis

_____ 3. iliopsoas

_____ 4. quadratus femoris

EXERCISE 10-11: COMPLETION

The vastus intermedius, lateralis, and medialis and rectus femoris form the _____.

EXERCISE 10-12: IDENTIFICATION

Identify the three muscles considered to make up the hamstring muscle.

A. _____

B. _____

C. _____

EXERCISE 10-13: IDENTIFICATION

Indicate whether the following muscles are (A) a flexor or (B) an extensor of the lower leg.

____ 1. gracilis

____ 2. hamstring

____ 3. quadriceps femoris

____ 4. sartorius

EXERCISE 10-14: IDENTIFICATION

Indicate which compartment the following muscles that move the foot are in: (A) anterior, (B) posterior, or (C) lateral.

____ 1. extensor digitorum longus

____ 2. flexor hallucis longus

____ 3. peroneus brevis

____ 4. popliteus

____ 5. soleus

EXERCISE 10-15: IDENTIFICATION

Identify the following items.

1. the thickest and strongest tendon in the human body

_____

2. the longest muscle in the human body

_____

3. the longest, heaviest, and strongest bone in the human body

_____

EXERCISE 10-16: LABELING

Label the following illustration from the list of terms provided.

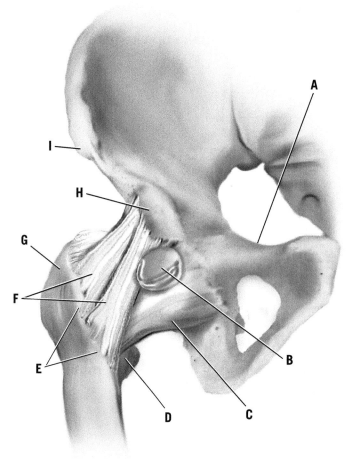

A. Anterior view

anterior inferior iliac spine
anterior superior iliac spine
greater trochanter
iliofemoral ligament
iliopectineal bursa
intertrochanteric line
lesser trochanter
pubofemoral ligament
superior pubic ramus

A. _____

B. _____

C. _____

D. _____

E. _____

F. _____

G. _____

H. _____

I. _____

EXERCISE 10-17: LABELING

Label the following illustration from the list of terms provided.

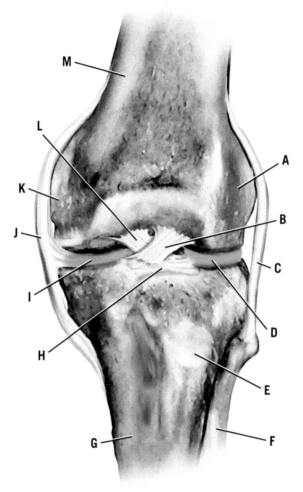

Ligaments of the knee: intracapsular, anterior view

anterior cruciate ligament

femur

fibula

fibular collateral ligament

lateral condyle of femur

lateral meniscus

medial condyle of femur

medial meniscus

posterior cruciate ligament

tibia

tibial collateral ligament

tibial tuberosity

transverse ligament

A. _____

B. _____

C. _____

D. _____

E. _____

F. _____

G. _____

H. _____

I. _____

J. _____

K. _____

L. _____

M. _____

EXERCISE 10-18: LABELING

Label the following illustration from the list of terms provided.

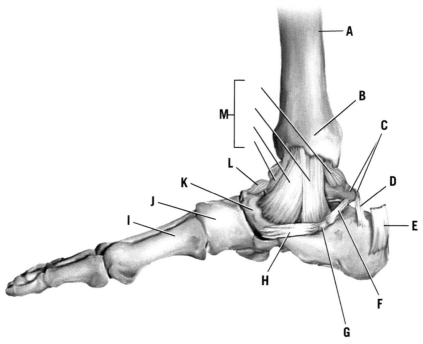

Copyright © 2015 Cengage Learning.®
Ligaments of the ankle, medial view

Achilles tendon (cut)
dorsal talonavicular ligament
first cuneiform bone
first metatarsal bone
medial (deltoid) ligament
medial malleolus of tibia
medial talocalcaneal ligament
navicular bone
plantar (spring) ligament
posterior process of talus
posterior talocalcaneal ligament
sustentaculum tali
tibia

A. _____
B. _____
C. _____
D. _____
E. _____
F. _____
G. _____
H. _____
I. _____
J. _____
K. _____
L. _____
M. _____

CT AXIAL IMAGES OF THE HIP

EXERCISE 10-19: LABELING

Label the following image from the list of terms provided in the Chapter 10 Word List in Appendix B.

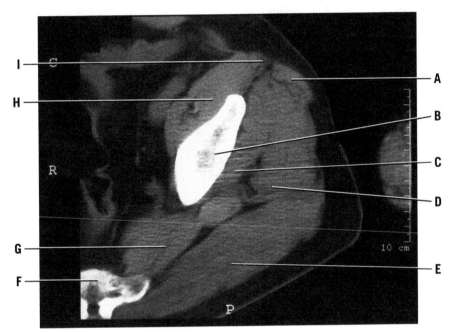

CT and MR Images provided by Roger Williams Medical Center.

A. _____

B. _____

C. _____

D. _____

E. _____

F. _____

G. _____

H. _____

I. _____

EXERCISE 10-20: LABELING

Label the following image from the list of terms provided in the Chapter 10 Word List in Appendix B.

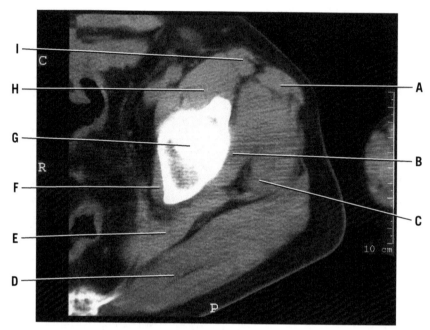

CT and MR Images provided by Roger Williams Medical Center.

A. _____

B. _____

C. _____

D. _____

E. _____

F. _____

G. _____

H. _____

I. _____

EXERCISE 10-21: LABELING

Label the following image from the list of terms provided in the Chapter 10 Word List in Appendix B.

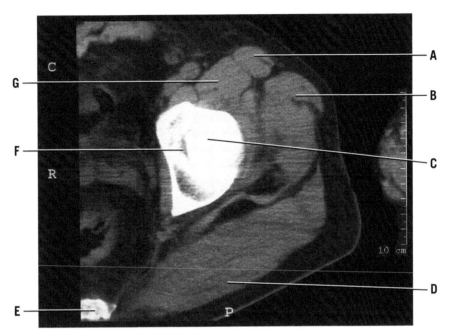

CT and MR Images provided by Roger Williams Medical Center.

A. _____

B. _____

C. _____

D. _____

E. _____

F. _____

G. _____

EXERCISE 10-22: LABELING

Label the following image from the list of terms provided in the Chapter 10 Word List in Appendix B.

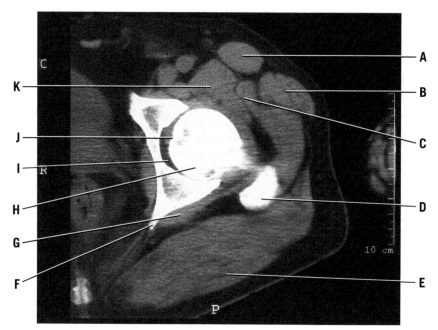

CT and MR Images provided by Roger Williams Medical Center.

A. _____

B. _____

C. _____

D. _____

E. _____

F. _____

G. _____

H. _____

I. _____

J. _____

K. _____

EXERCISE 10-23: LABELING

Label the following image from the list of terms provided in the Chapter 10 Word List in Appendix B.

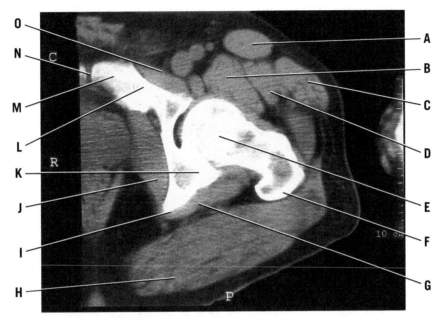

CT and MR Images provided by Roger Williams Medical Center.

A. _____

B. _____

C. _____

D. _____

E. _____

F. _____

G. _____

H. _____

I. _____

J. _____

K. _____

L. _____

M. _____

N. _____

O. _____

EXERCISE 10-24: LABELING

Label the following image from the list of terms provided in the Chapter 10 Word List in Appendix B.

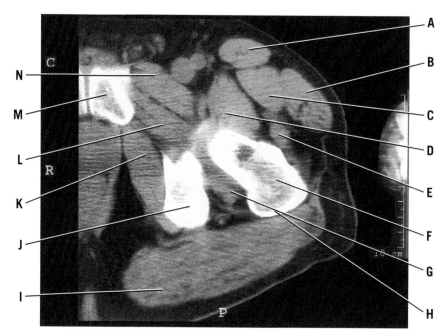

CT and MR Images provided by Roger Williams Medical Center.

A. _____

B. _____

C. _____

D. _____

E. _____

F. _____

G. _____

H. _____

I. _____

J. _____

K. _____

L. _____

M. _____

N. _____

EXERCISE 10-25: LABELING

Label the following image from the list of terms provided in the Chapter 10 Word List in Appendix B.

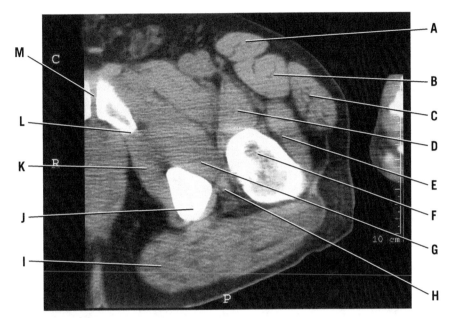

CT and MR Images provided by Roger Williams Medical Center.

A. _____

B. _____

C. _____

D. _____

E. _____

F. _____

G. _____

H. _____

I. _____

J. _____

K. _____

L. _____

M. _____

EXERCISE 10-26: LABELING

Label the following image from the list of terms provided in the Chapter 10 Word List in Appendix B.

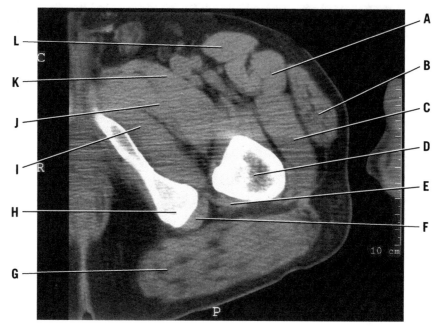

CT and MR Images provided by Roger Williams Medical Center.

A. _____

B. _____

C. _____

D. _____

E. _____

F. _____

G. _____

H. _____

I. _____

J. _____

K. _____

L. _____

MR IMAGES OF THE HIP

AXIAL IMAGES

EXERCISE 10-27: LABELING

Label the following image from the list of terms provided in the Chapter 10 Word List in Appendix B.

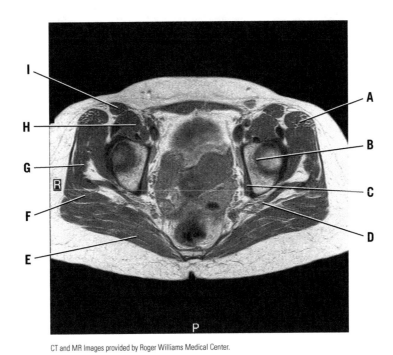

CT and MR Images provided by Roger Williams Medical Center.

A. _____

B. _____

C. _____

D. _____

E. _____

F. _____

G. _____

H. _____

I. _____

EXERCISE 10-28: LABELING

Label the following image from the list of terms provided in the Chapter 10 Word List in Appendix B.

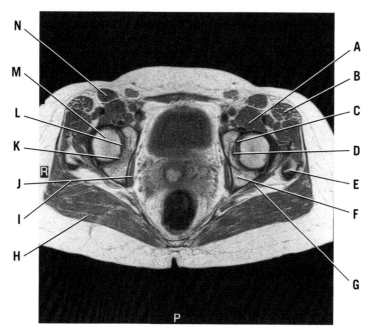

CT and MR Images provided by Roger Williams Medical Center.

A. _____

B. _____

C. _____

D. _____

E. _____

F. _____

G. _____

H. _____

I. _____

J. _____

K. _____

L. _____

M. _____

N. _____

EXERCISE 10-29: LABELING

Label the following image from the list of terms provided in the Chapter 10 Word List in Appendix B.

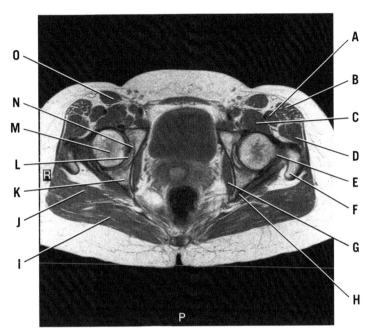

CT and MR Images provided by Roger Williams Medical Center.

A. _____   I. _____

B. _____   J. _____

C. _____   K. _____

D. _____   L. _____

E. _____   M. _____

F. _____   N. _____

G. _____   O. _____

H. _____

EXERCISE 10-30: LABELING

Label the following image from the list of terms provided in the Chapter 10 Word List in Appendix B.

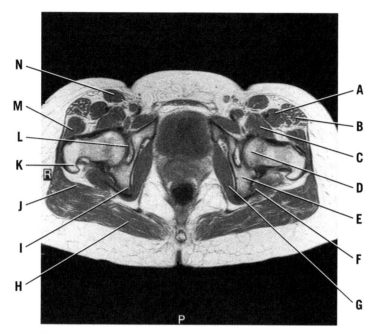

CT and MR Images provided by Roger Williams Medical Center.

A. _____

B. _____

C. _____

D. _____

E. _____

F. _____

G. _____

H. _____

I. _____

J. _____

K. _____

L. _____

M. _____

N. _____

CORONAL IMAGES

EXERCISE 10-31: LABELING

Label the following image from the list of terms provided in the Chapter 10 Word List in Appendix B.

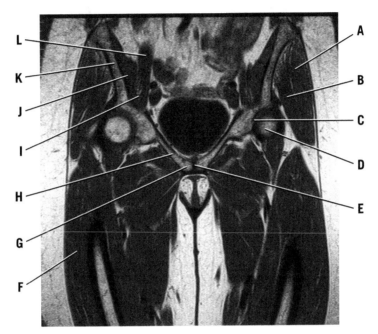

CT and MR Images provided by Roger Williams Medical Center.

A. _____

B. _____

C. _____

D. _____

E. _____

F. _____

G. _____

H. _____

I. _____

J. _____

K. _____

L. _____

EXERCISE 10-32: LABELING

Label the following image from the list of terms provided in the Chapter 10 Word List in Appendix B.

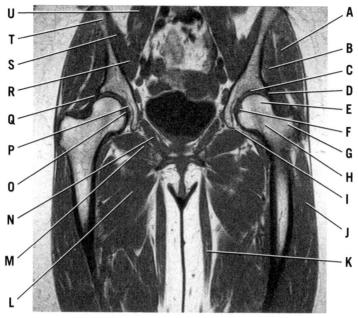

CT and MR Images provided by Roger Williams Medical Center.

A. _____   L. _____

B. _____   M. _____

C. _____   N. _____

D. _____   O. _____

E. _____   P. _____

F. _____   Q. _____

G. _____   R. _____

H. _____   S. _____

I. _____   T. _____

J. _____   U. _____

K. _____

EXERCISE 10-33: LABELING

Label the following image from the list of terms provided in the Chapter 10 Word List in Appendix B.

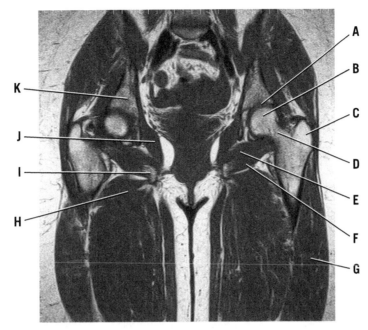

CT and MR Images provided by Roger Williams Medical Center.

A. _____

B. _____

C. _____

D. _____

E. _____

F. _____

G. _____

H. _____

I. _____

J. _____

K. _____

SAGITTAL IMAGES

EXERCISE 10-34: LABELING

Label the following image from the list of terms provided in the Chapter 10 Word List in Appendix B.

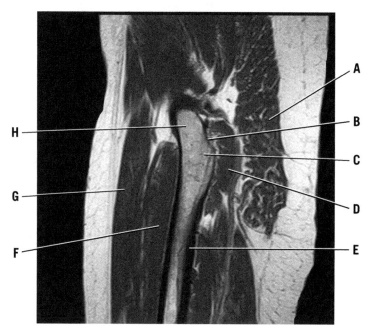

CT and MR Images provided by Roger Williams Medical Center.

A. _____

B. _____

C. _____

D. _____

E. _____

F. _____

G. _____

H. _____

EXERCISE 10-35: LABELING

Label the following image from the list of terms provided in the Chapter 10 Word List in Appendix B.

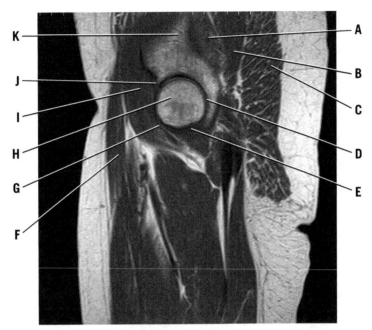

CT and MR Images provided by Roger Williams Medical Center.

A. _____

B. _____

C. _____

D. _____

E. _____

F. _____

G. _____

H. _____

I. _____

J. _____

K. _____

CT AXIAL IMAGES OF THE KNEE

EXERCISE 10-36: LABELING

Label the following image from the list of terms provided in the Chapter 10 Word List in Appendix B.

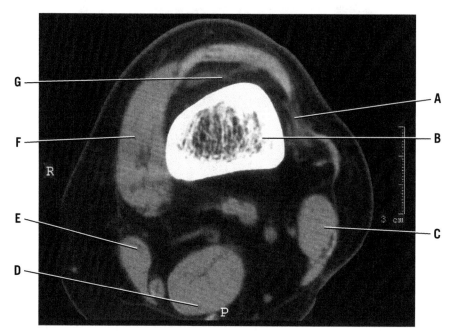

CT and MR Images provided by Roger Williams Medical Center.

A. _____

B. _____

C. _____

D. _____

E. _____

F. _____

G. _____

EXERCISE 10-37: LABELING

Label the following image from the list of terms provided in the Chapter 10 Word List in Appendix B.

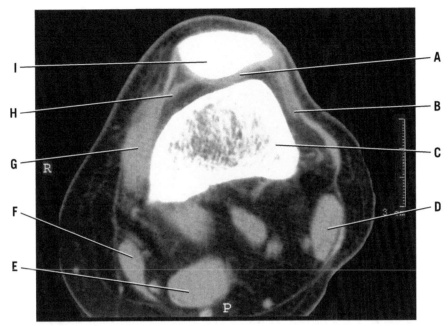

CT and MR Images provided by Roger Williams Medical Center.

A. _____

B. _____

C. _____

D. _____

E. _____

F. _____

G. _____

H. _____

I. _____

EXERCISE 10-38: LABELING

Label the following image from the list of terms provided in the Chapter 10 Word List in Appendix B.

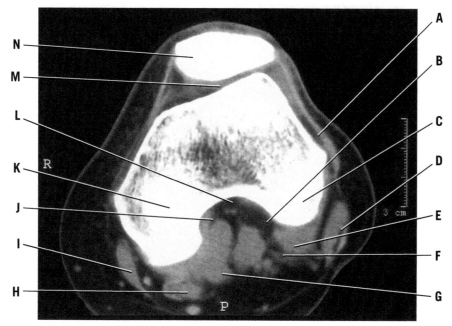

CT and MR Images provided by Roger Williams Medical Center.

A. _____

B. _____

C. _____

D. _____

E. _____

F. _____

G. _____

H. _____

I. _____

J. _____

K. _____

L. _____

M. _____

N. _____

EXERCISE 10-39: LABELING

Label the following image from the list of terms provided in the Chapter 10 Word List in Appendix B.

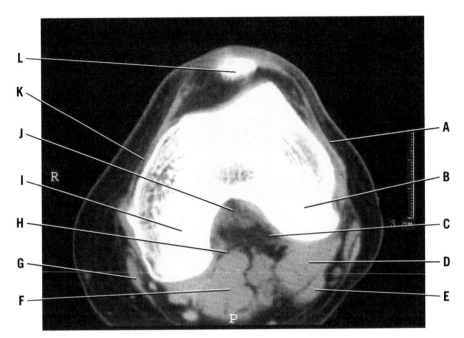

CT and MR Images provided by Roger Williams Medical Center.

A. _____

B. _____

C. _____

D. _____

E. _____

F. _____

G. _____

H. _____

I. _____

J. _____

K. _____

L. _____

EXERCISE 10-40: LABELING

Label the following image from the list of terms provided in the Chapter 10 Word List in Appendix B.

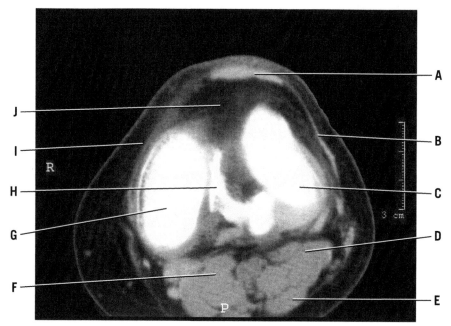

CT and MR Images provided by Roger Williams Medical Center.

A. _____

B. _____

C. _____

D. _____

E. _____

F. _____

G. _____

H. _____

I. _____

J. _____

EXERCISE 10-41: LABELING

Label the following image from the list of terms provided in the Chapter 10 Word List in Appendix B.

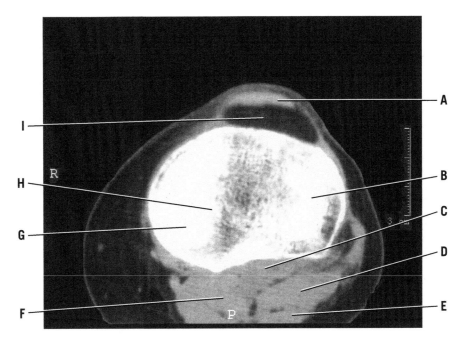

CT and MR Images provided by Roger Williams Medical Center.

A. _____

B. _____

C. _____

D. _____

E. _____

F. _____

G. _____

H. _____

I. _____

EXERCISE 10-42: LABELING

Label the following image from the list of terms provided in the Chapter 10 Word List in Appendix B.

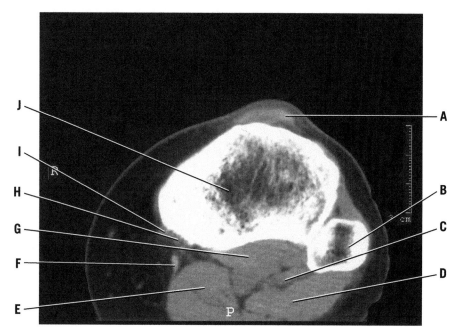

CT and MR Images provided by Roger Williams Medical Center.

A. _____

B. _____

C. _____

D. _____

E. _____

F. _____

G. _____

H. _____

I. _____

J. _____

MR IMAGES OF THE KNEE

AXIAL IMAGE

EXERCISE 10-43: LABELING

Label the following image from the list of terms provided in the Chapter 10 Word List in Appendix B.

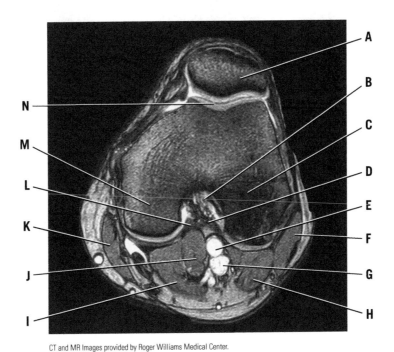

CT and MR Images provided by Roger Williams Medical Center.

A. _____   H. _____

B. _____   I. _____

C. _____   J. _____

D. _____   K. _____

E. _____   L. _____

F. _____   M. _____

G. _____   N. _____

CORONAL IMAGES

EXERCISE 10-44: LABELING

Label the following image from the list of terms provided in the Chapter 10 Word List in Appendix B.

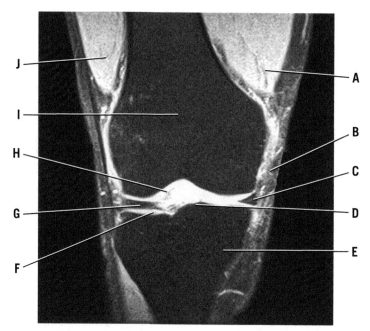

CT and MR Images provided by Roger Williams Medical Center.

A. _____

B. _____

C. _____

D. _____

E. _____

F. _____

G. _____

H. _____

I. _____

J. _____

EXERCISE 10-45: LABELING

Label the following image from the list of terms provided in the Chapter 10 Word List in Appendix B.

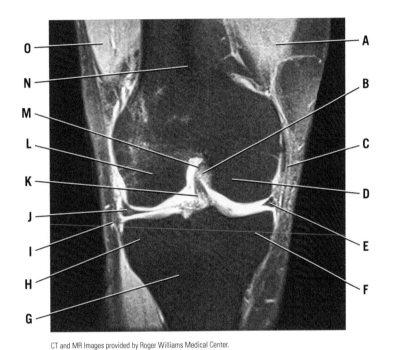

CT and MR Images provided by Roger Williams Medical Center.

A. _____   I. _____

B. _____   J. _____

C. _____   K. _____

D. _____   L. _____

E. _____   M. _____

F. _____   N. _____

G. _____   O. _____

H. _____

SAGITTAL IMAGES

EXERCISE 10-46: LABELING

Label the following image from the list of terms provided in the **Chapter 10 Word List in Appendix B.**

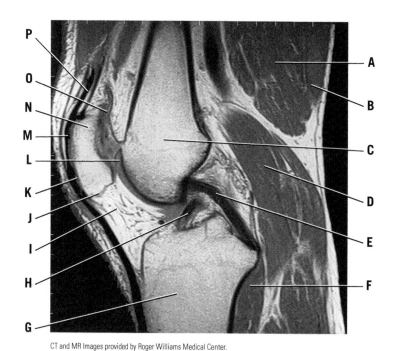

CT and MR Images provided by Roger Williams Medical Center.

A. _____   I. _____

B. _____   J. _____

C. _____   K. _____

D. _____   L. _____

E. _____   M. _____

F. _____   N. _____

G. _____   O. _____

H. _____   P. _____

EXERCISE 10-47: LABELING

Label the following image from the list of terms provided in the Chapter 10 Word List in Appendix B.

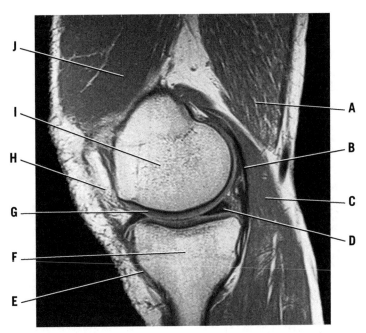

CT and MR Images provided by Roger Williams Medical Center.

A. _____

B. _____

C. _____

D. _____

E. _____

F. _____

G. _____

H. _____

I. _____

J. _____

CT AXIAL IMAGES OF THE ANKLE

EXERCISE 10-48: LABELING

Label the following image from the list of terms provided in the Chapter 10 Word List in Appendix B.

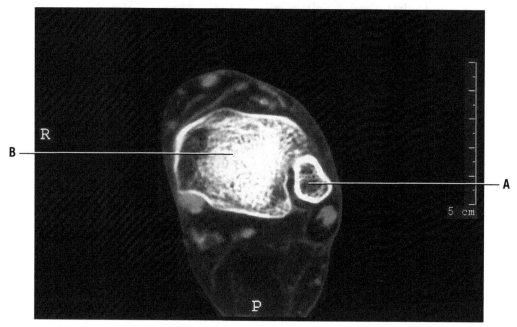

CT and MR Images provided by Roger Williams Medical Center.

A. _____

B. _____

EXERCISE 10-49: LABELING

Label the following image from the list of terms provided in the Chapter 10 Word List in Appendix B.

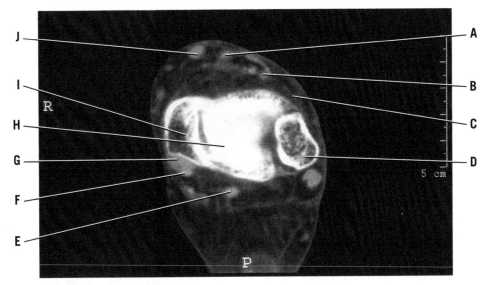

CT and MR Images provided by Roger Williams Medical Center.

A. _____

B. _____

C. _____

D. _____

E. _____

F. _____

G. _____

H. _____

I. _____

J. _____

EXERCISE 10-50: LABELING

Label the following image from the list of terms provided in the Chapter 10 Word List in Appendix B.

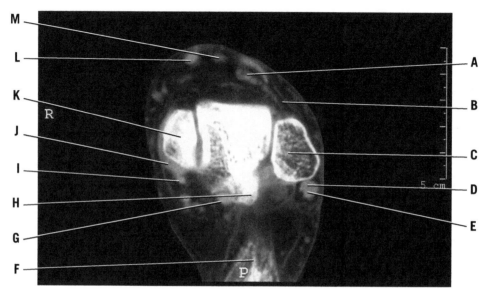

CT and MR Images provided by Roger Williams Medical Center.

A. _____

B. _____

C. _____

D. _____

E. _____

F. _____

G. _____

H. _____

I. _____

J. _____

K. _____

L. _____

M. _____

EXERCISE 10-51: LABELING

Label the following image from the list of terms provided in the Chapter 10 Word List in Appendix B.

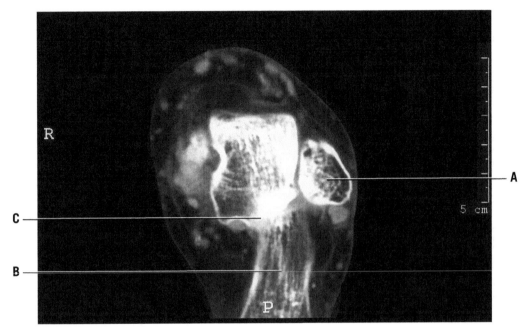

CT and MR Images provided by Roger Williams Medical Center.

A. _____

B. _____

C. _____

EXERCISE 10-52: LABELING

Label the following image from the list of terms provided in the Chapter 10 Word List in Appendix B.

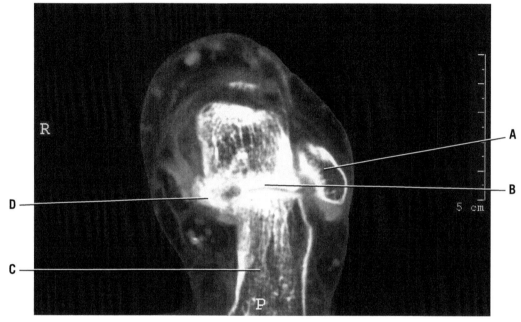

CT and MR Images provided by Roger Williams Medical Center.

A. _____

B. _____

C. _____

D. _____

EXERCISE 10-53: LABELING

Label the following image from the list of terms provided in the Chapter 10 Word List in Appendix B.

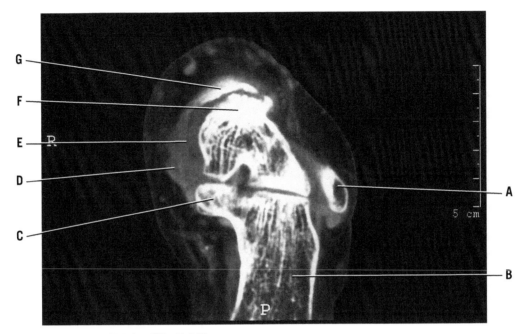

CT and MR Images provided by Roger Williams Medical Center.

A. _____

B. _____

C. _____

D. _____

E. _____

F. _____

G. _____

EXERCISE 10-54: LABELING

Label the following image from the list of terms provided in the Chapter 10 Word List in Appendix B.

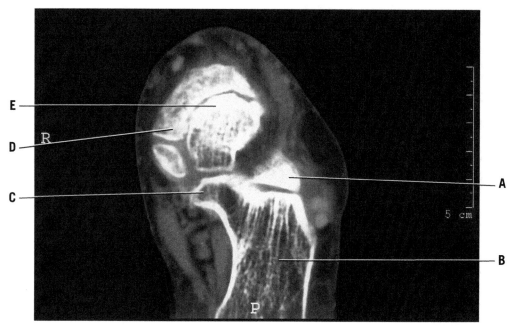

CT and MR Images provided by Roger Williams Medical Center.

A. _____

B. _____

C. _____

D. _____

E. _____

EXERCISE 10-55: LABELING

Label the following image from the list of terms provided in the Chapter 10 Word List in Appendix B.

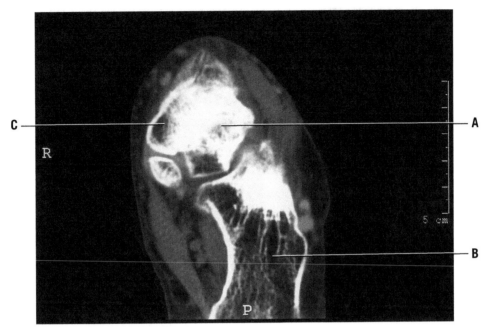

CT and MR Images provided by Roger Williams Medical Center.

A. _____

B. _____

C. _____

EXERCISE 10-56: LABELING

Label the following image from the list of terms provided in the Chapter 10 Word List in Appendix B.

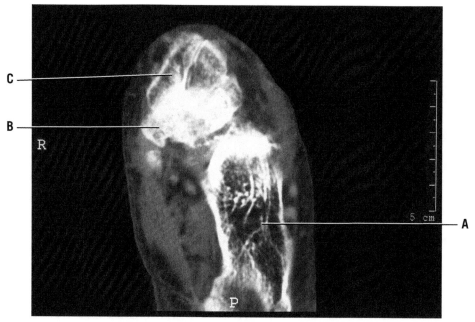

CT and MR Images provided by Roger Williams Medical Center.

A. _____

B. _____

C. _____

EXERCISE 10-57: LABELING

Label the following image from the list of terms provided in the Chapter 10 Word List in Appendix B.

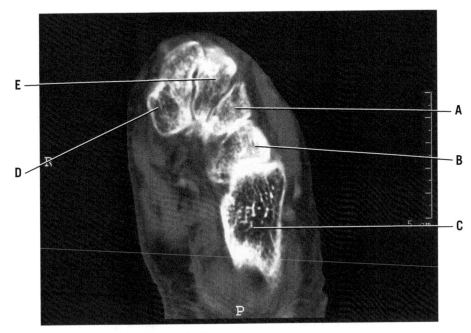

CT and MR Images provided by Roger Williams Medical Center.

A. _____

B. _____

C. _____

D. _____

E. _____

MR IMAGES OF THE ANKLE

AXIAL IMAGE

EXERCISE 10-58: LABELING

Label the following image from the list of terms provided in the Chapter 10 Word List in Appendix B.

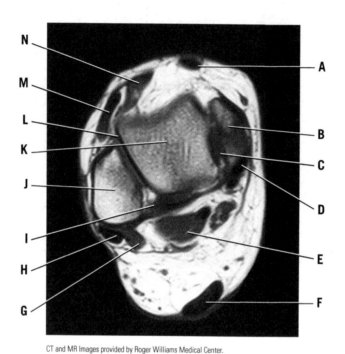

CT and MR Images provided by Roger Williams Medical Center.

A. _____   H. _____

B. _____   I. _____

C. _____   J. _____

D. _____   K. _____

E. _____   L. _____

F. _____   M. _____

G. _____   N. _____

CORONAL IMAGE

EXERCISE 10-59: LABELING

Label the following image from the list of terms provided in the **Chapter 10 Word List** in Appendix B.

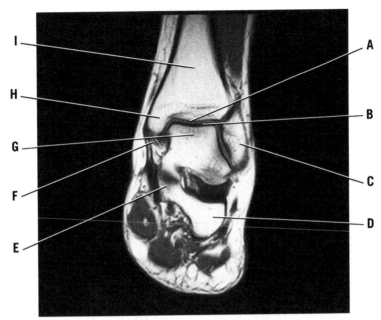

CT and MR Images provided by Roger Williams Medical Center.

A. _____

B. _____

C. _____

D. _____

E. _____

F. _____

G. _____

H. _____

I. _____

SAGITTAL IMAGES

EXERCISE 10-60: LABELING

Label the following image from the list of terms provided in the Chapter 10 Word List in Appendix B.

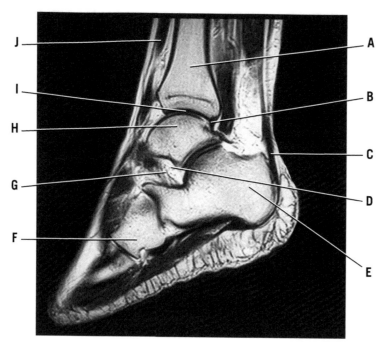

CT and MR Images provided by Roger Williams Medical Center.

A. _____

B. _____

C. _____

D. _____

E. _____

F. _____

G. _____

H. _____

I. _____

J. _____

EXERCISE 10-61: LABELING

Label the following image from the list of terms provided in the Chapter 10 Word List in Appendix B.

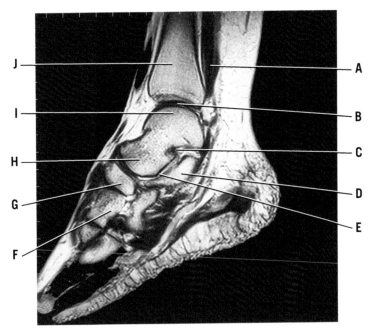

CT and MR Images provided by Roger Williams Medical Center.

A. _____

B. _____

C. _____

D. _____

E. _____

F. _____

G. _____

H. _____

I. _____

J. _____

Appendix A
Answer Key

CHAPTER 1: INTRODUCTION

Exercise 1-1: Matching

A. proximal
B. distal
C. medial
D. lateral
E. distal
F. proximal
G. inferior (caudal)
H. posterior (dorsal)
I. anterior (ventral)
J. superior (cephalad)

Exercise 1-2: Labeling

A. cranial cavity
B. dorsal cavity
C. spinal cavity
D. pelvic cavity
E. abdominopelvic cavity
F. division between abdominal and pelvic cavities
G. abdominal cavity
H. ventral cavity
I. diaphragm
J. thoracic cavity

Exercise 1-3: Labeling

A. midcoronal plane
B. transverse plane
C. midsagittal plane

Exercise 1-4: Labeling

A. epigastric region
B. left hypochondriac region
C. left lumbar region
D. left inguinal region
E. hypogastric region
F. right inguinal region
G. umbilical region
H. right lumbar region
I. right hypochondriac region

Exercise 1-5: Matching

1. C
2. B
3. D
4. A

Exercise 1-6: Identification

1. A
2. B
3. B
4. A
5. A
6. A
7. B
8. A
9. B
10. B
11. A
12. B
13. A

CHAPTER 2: HEAD

Exercise 2-1: Matching

1. h
2. f
3. d
4. b
5. g
6. j
7. i
8. a
9. e
10. c

Exercise 2-2: Term Identification

1. foramina of Luschka
2. interventricular foramen or foramen of Monro
3. foramen of Magendie
4. cerebral aqueduct or aqueduct of Sylvius

Exercise 2-3: Completion

(Terms listed in the order they appear.)
cerebrum
diencephalon
cortex
gray
centrum semiovale
white
gray
longitudinal

corpus callosum
central
lateral (Sylvian)
tranverse
thalamus
hypothalamus
thalamus
hypothalamus
infundibulum
peduncles
quadrigeminal plate
cerebral aqueduct
pons
medulla oblongata
cerebellum
cerebellum
vermis
medulla oblongata
spinal cord
midbrain
pons
medulla oblongata

Exercise 2-4: Labeling

A. choroid plexus of third ventricle
B. body of corpus callosum
C. intermediate mass of thalamus
D. choroid plexus of lateral ventricle
E. lateral ventricle (anterior horn)
F. corpus callosum
G. fornix
H. foramen of Monro
I. genu of corpus callosum
J. peduncles
K. cerebrum
L. infundibulum
M. pituitary gland
N. cerebral aqueduct
O. pons
P. cistern pontine
Q. medulla oblongata
R. spinal cord
S. cisterna magna
T. central canal
U. foramen of Magendie
V. fourth ventricle
W. choroid plexus of fourth ventricle

X. skull
Y. cerebellum
Z. quadrigeminal plate
AA. quadrigeminal cistern
BB. splenium of corpus callosum
CC. pineal gland
DD. third ventricle
EE. pia mater
FF. subarachnoid space
GG. arachnoid
HH. subdural space
II. dura mater

Exercise 2-5: Labeling

A. left common carotid artery
B. left vertebral artery
C. left subclavian artery
D. ascending aorta
E. arch of aorta
F. brachiocephalic (innominate) artery
G. right subclavian artery
H. right vertebral artery
I. right common carotid artery
J. right external carotid artery
K. right internal carotid artery

Exercise 2-6: Labeling

A. superior sagittal sinus
B. sulcus
C. left hemisphere of cerebrum
D. gyrus
E. longitudinal fissure
F. right hemisphere of cerebrum
G. white matter
H. cranium

Exercise 2-7: Labeling

A. frontal lobe of cerebrum
B. falx cerebri
C. parietal lobe of cerebrum

Exercise 2-8: Labeling

A. cortex—gray matter
B. body of corpus callosum
C. left hemisphere of cerebrum
D. longitudinal fissure
E. centrum semiovale—white matter
F. right hemisphere of cerebrum

Exercise 2-9: Labeling

A. gyrus
B. corpus callosum
C. cortex
D. occipital lobe of cerebrum
E. sulcus
F. cranium

Exercise 2-10: Labeling

A. genu of corpus callosum
B. body of lateral ventricle
C. splenium of corpus callosum
D. septum pellucidum

Exercise 2-.11: Labeling

A. genu of corpus callosum
B. body of lateral ventricle
C. longitudinal fissure
D. splenium of corpus callosum
E. septum pellucidum

Exercise 2-12: Labeling

A. head of caudate nucleus
B. posterior horn of lateral ventricle
C. centrum semiovale
D. anterior horn of lateral ventricle

Exercise 2-13: Labeling

A. anterior horn of lateral ventricle
B. collateral trigone
C. posterior horn of lateral ventricle
D. head of caudate nucleus

Exercise 2-14: Labeling

A. head of caudate nucleus
B. putamen
C. interventricular foramen
D. third ventricle
E. collateral trigone—choroid plexus
F. pineal gland
G. thalamus
H. globus pallidus
I. internal capsule

Exercise 2-15: Labeling

A. Sylvian or lateral fissure
B. parietal lobe of cerebrum
C. third ventricle
D. pineal gland
E. thalamus
F. frontal lobe of cerebrum

Exercise 2-16: Labeling

A. insula or central lobe of cerebrum
B. Sylvian or lateral fissure

Exercise 2-17: Labeling

A. quadrigeminal plate
B. aqueduct of Sylvius
C. quadrigeminal cistern
D. peduncle

Exercise 2-18: Labeling

A. middle cerebral artery
B. pons
C. left hemisphere of cerebellum
D. right hemisphere of cerebellum
E. vermis
F. tentorium cerebelli
G. fourth ventricle
H. posterior cerebral artery

Exercise 2-19: Labeling

A. anterior clinoid of sphenoid bone
B. pituitary gland in sella turcica
C. dorsum sellae
D. fourth ventricle
E. left hemisphere of cerebellum
F. right hemisphere of cerebellum
G. pons
H. posterior clinoids of sphenoid bone
I. temporal lobe of cerebrum

Exercise 2-20: Labeling

A. temporal lobe of cerebrum
B. fourth ventricle
C. cerebellum
D. petrous ridge

Exercise 2-21: Labeling

A. gyrus
B. centrum semiovale

C. cranium
D. parietal lobe of cerebrum
E. scalp
F. sulcus
G. cortex—gray matter
H. longitudinal fissure
I. frontal lobe of cerebrum
J. diploë

Exercise 2-22: Labeling

A. anterior superior sagittal sinus
B. body of corpus callosum
C. posterior superior sagittal sinus
D. lateral ventricle

Exercise 2-23: Labeling

A. genu of corpus callosum
B. septum pellucidum
C. splenium of corpus callosum
D. occipital lobe of cerebrum
E. body of lateral ventricle

Exercise 2-24: Labeling

A. anterior horn of lateral ventricle
B. internal capsule
C. interventricular foramen
D. third ventricle
E. thalamus
F. posterior horn of lateral ventricle
G. globus pallidus
H. lentiform nucleus
I. putamen
J. corpus striatum
K. head of caudate nucleus

Exercise 2-25: Labeling

A. head of caudate nucleus
B. choroid plexus in collateral trigone
C. anterior horn of lateral ventricle
D. longitudinal fissure

Exercise 2-26: Labeling

A. frontal lobe of cerebrum
B. Sylvian or lateral fissure
C. third ventricle
D. thalamus

E. central lobe or insula of cerebrum
F. longitudinal fissure

Exercise 2-27: Labeling

A. Sylvian or lateral fissure
B. central lobe or insula of cerebrum

Exercise 2-28: Labeling

A. peduncle
B. aqueduct of Sylvius (cerebral aqueduct)
C. quadrigeminal cistern
D. quadrigeminal plate

Exercise 2-29: Labeling

A. aqueduct of Sylvius (cerebral aqueduct)
B. vermis
C. transverse fissure
D. quadrigeminal plate
E. midbrain
F. peduncle

Exercise 2-30: Labeling

A. pons
B. tentorium cerebelli
C. left hemisphere of cerebellum
D. right hemisphere of cerebellum
E. fourth ventricle
F. basilar artery

Exercise 2-31: Labeling

A. petrous pyramid
B. cerebellum
C. falx cerebelli
D. fourth ventricle
E. pons
F. temporal lobe of cerebrum

Exercise 2-32: Labeling

A. internal carotid artery
B. cerebellum
C. falx cerebelli
D. petrous pyramid

Exercise 2-33: Labeling

A. parietal lobe of cerebrum
B. cortex

C. cranium
D. gyrus
E. third ventricle
F. splenium of corpus callosum
G. occipital lobe of cerebrum
H. quadrigeminal cistern
I. transverse fissure
J. scalp
K. thalamus
L. cerebellum (vermis)
M. anterior cerebellar notch
N. fourth ventricle
O. cisterna magna
P. foramen of Magendie
Q. spinal cord
R. medulla
S. cistern pontine
T. pons
U. pituitary gland
V. quadrigeminal plate
W. midbrain
X. peduncles
Y. optic nerve
Z. optic chiasma
AA. cerebral aqueduct
BB. hypothalamus
CC. anterior horn of lateral ventricle
DD. genu of corpus callosum
EE. frontal lobe of cerebrum
FF. sulcus
GG. fornix
HH. body of corpus callosum

Exercise 2-34: Labeling

A. fat—scalp
B. cranium
C. longitudinal fissure
D. left hemisphere of cerebrum
E. white matter
F. sulcus
G. gyrus
H. cortex—gray matter
I. frontal lobe of cerebrum
J. right hemisphere of cerebrum

Exercise 2-35: Labeling

A. scalp
B. frontal lobe of cerebrum
C. genu of corpus callosum
D. gyrus

E. left hemisphere of cerebrum
F. right hemisphere of cerebrum
G. sulcus
H. cortex
I. cranium
J. longitudinal fissure (falx cerebri)

Exercise 2-36: Labeling

A. white matter – centrum semiovale
B. head of caudate nucleus
C. septum pellucidum
D. lentiform nucleus
E. optic chiasma
F. internal carotid artery
G. pituitary gland
H. infundibulum
I. internal capsule
J. insula
K. Sylvian fissure
L. anterior horn of lateral ventricle
M. body of corpus callosum
N. cortex – gray matter

Exercise 2-37: Labeling

A. parietal lobe of cerebrum
B. head of caudate nucleus
C. septum pellucidum
D. Sylvian fissure
E. insula (central lobe) of cerebrum
F. third ventricle
G. thalamus
H. globus pallidus
I. lentiform nucleus
J. putamen
K. interventricular foramen
L. internal capsule
M. anterior horn - lateral ventricle
N. body of corpus callosum

Exercise 2-38: Labeling

A. falx cerebri
B. lateral fissure
C. third ventricle
D. pons
E. centrum semiovale

Exercise 2-39: Labeling

A. corpus callosum
B. Sylvian fissure
C. third ventricle
D. pons
E. central lobe or insula of cerebrum
F. lateral ventricle
G. longitudinal fissure

Exercise 2-40: Labeling

A. third ventricle
B. Sylvian fissure
C. superior colliculus
D. inferior colliculus
E. tentorium cerebelli
F. medulla oblongata
G. cerebral peduncle
H. cerebellum
I. cerebral aqueduct
J. temporal lobe of cerebrum
K. body of lateral ventricle

Exercise 2-41: Labeling

A. superior sagittal sinus
B. cerebrum
C. pineal gland
D. transverse fissure
E. fourth ventricle
F. foramen of Luschka (lateral apertures)
G. median aperture
H. cerebellum
I. tentorium cerebelli
J. quadrigeminal cistern
K. collateral trigone

Exercise 2-42: Labeling

A. white matter
B. splenium of corpus callosum
C. white matter
D. cisterna magna
E. falx cerebelli
F. posterior horn of lateral ventricle

Exercise 2-43: Labeling

A. gyrus
B. sulcus
C. occipital horn of lateral ventricle

D. tentorium cerebelli—transverse fissure
E. left hemisphere of cerebellum
F. cisterna magna
G. right hemisphere of cerebellum
H. occipital lobe of cerebrum
I. falx cerebri—longitudinal fissure

Exercise 2-44: Labeling

A. longitudinal fissure
B. left hemisphere of cerebrum
C. white matter
D. tentorium cerebelli
E. left hemisphere of cerebellum
F. right hemisphere of cerebellum
G. vermis
H. right hemisphere of cerebrum
I. sulcus
J. gyrus

Exercise 2-45: Labeling

A. scalp
B. falx cerebri—longitudinal fissure
C. left hemisphere of cerebrum
D. left hemisphere of cerebellum
E. right hemisphere of cerebellum
F. right hemisphere of cerebrum
G. cranium

Exercise 2-46: Labeling

A. cortex—gray matter
B. left hemisphere of cerebrum
C. cerebellum
D. right hemisphere of cerebrum
E. falx cerebri

Exercise 2-47: Labeling

A. cortex
B. longitudinal fissure
C. left hemisphere of cerebrum
D. occipital lobe of cerebrum
E. right hemisphere of cerebrum

CHAPTER 3: FACE

Exercise 3-1: Labeling

A. ethmoid—crista galli
B. ethmoid cribriform plate
C. sphenoid sella turcica

D. sphenoid sinus
E. sphenoid bone
F. lateral pterygoid process of sphenoid bone
G. medial pterygoid process of sphenoid bone
H. perpendicular plate of palatine bone
I. horizontal plate of palatine bone
J. palatine process of maxilla
K. vomer
L. septal cartilage
M. ethmoid perpendicular plate
N. nasal bone
O. frontal sinus
P. frontal bone

Exercise 3-2: Matching

1. b
2. c
3. a
4. d

Exercise 3-3: Identification

1. frontal
2. maxillary
3. zygomatic
4. ethmoid
5. lacrimal
6. sphenoid
7. palatine

Exercise 3-4: Identification

1. maxillary
2. frontal
3. ethmoid
4. sphenoid

Exercise 3-5: Completion

(Terms listed in the order they appear.)
maxillary
ethmoid
frontal
maxillary
maxillary

Exercise 3-6: Labeling

A. frontal sinus
B. nasal bone

C. frontal process of maxillary bone
D. perpendicular plate of ethmoid bone
E. frontal bone

Exercise 3-7: Labeling

A. frontal sinus
B. lacrimal bone
C. alveolar process of maxillary bone
D. perpendicular plate of ethmoid bone
E. superior orbital margin
F. frontal bone

Exercise 3-8: Labeling

A. superior orbital margin
B. lateral mass of ethmoid bone
C. zygoma
D. maxillary sinus
E. inferior nasal concha
F. mentum of mandible
G. vomer
H. maxillary bone
I. inferior orbital margin
J. middle nasal concha
K. ethmoidal air cells
L. cribriform plate of ethmoid bone
M. crista galli

Exercise 3-9: Labeling

A. superior orbital margin (frontal bone)
B. crista galli
C. zygomatic (malar) bone
D. vomer
E. inferior nasal concha
F. maxillary sinus
G. middle nasal concha
H. superior nasal concha
I. lateral mass of ethmoid bone
J. ethmoid sinus
K. cribriform plate

Exercise 3-10: Labeling

A. optic nerve
B. lateral rectus muscle
C. maxillary sinus
D. mandible

E. vomer
F. inferior rectus muscle
G. medial rectus muscle
H. superior rectus muscle

Exercise 3-11: Labeling

A. perpendicular plate of ethmoid bone
B. maxillary sinus
C. inferior nasal concha
D. vomer
E. middle nasal concha
F. sphenoid bone
G. cribriform plate of ethmoid bone

Exercise 3-12: Labeling

A. anterior clinoid
B. sphenoid sinus
C. maxillary sinus
D. body of sphenoid

Exercise 3-13: Labeling

A. frontal sinus
B. diploë
C. compact bone
D. frontal bone

Exercise 3-14: Labeling

A. roof of orbit formed by horizontal portion of frontal bone

Exercise 3-15: Labeling

A. lateral mass of ethmoid bone

Exercise 3-16: Labeling

A. nasal bone
B. perpendicular plate of ethmoid bone
C. medial rectus muscle
D. lateral rectus muscle
E. optic nerve
F. ethmoidal air cells
G. lens of eye

Exercise 3-17: Labeling

A. lacrimal bone
B. ethmoidal air cells
C. sphenoid sinus

D. zygoma
E. bony nasal septum

Exercise 3-18: Labeling

A. maxillary bone
B. zygoma
C. sphenoid sinus
D. nasal concha
E. maxillary sinus
F. bony nasal septum

Exercise 3-19: Labeling

A. zygoma
B. bony nasal septum
C. sphenoid sinus
D. temporal bone
E. mastoid air cells
F. maxillary sinus

Exercise 3-20: Labeling

A. maxillary sinus

Exercise 3-21: Labeling

A. palatine bone
B. mandible
C. palatine processes of maxillary bone

Exercise 3-22: Labeling

A. mandible
B. alveolar process of maxillary bone

CHAPTER 4: NECK

Exercise 4-1: Labeling

A. sternohyoid muscle
B. sternocleidomastoid (SCM) muscle
C. clavicle
D. first rib
E. sternothyroid muscle
F. posterior scalene muscle
G. middle scalene muscle
H. anterior scalene muscle
I. thyroid cartilage
J. hyoid bone

Exercise 4-2: Matching

1. c
2. d
3. e
4. a
5. b

Exercise 4-3: Identification

1. sublingual
2. parotid
3. submandibular

Exercise 4-4: Identification

1. nasopharynx
2. oropharynx
3. laryngopharynx

Exercise 4-5: Completion

(Terms listed in the order they appear.)
laryngo-
trachea
esophagus
cricoid cartilage
C5/C6
trachea
right and left primary bronchi
T4/T5
esophagus

Exercise 4-6: Labeling

A. epiglottis
B. hyoid bone
C. thyroid cartilage
D. corniculate cartilage
E. arytenoid cartilage
F. vocal cords
G. cricoid cartilage
H. trachea

Exercise 4-7: Labeling

A. mandible
B. longus capitis/longus colli muscle
C. internal carotid artery
D. sternocleidomastoid muscle (SCM)
E. internal jugular vein
F. anterior, middle, posterior scalene muscles

G. erector spinae muscle
H. vertebral artery
I. external jugular vein
J. external carotid artery
K. platysma
L. pharynx

Exercise 4-8: Labeling

A. epiglottis
B. submandibular gland
C. anterior jugular vein
D. left common carotid artery
E. longus capitis/longus colli muscles
F. vertebral artery
G. erector spinae muscle
H. scalene muscles
I. SCM
J. external jugular vein
K. right internal carotid artery
L. right external carotid artery
M. hyoid bone
N. pharynx
O. platysma

Exercise 4-9: Labeling

A. submandibular gland
B. anterior jugular vein
C. common carotid artery
D. internal jugular vein
E. erector spinae muscle
F. scalene muscles
G. external jugular vein
H. SCM
I. pharynx
J. hyoid bone
K. platysma

Exercise 4-10: Labeling

A. platysma
B. pharynx
C. anterior jugular vein
D. SCM
E. internal jugular vein
F. longus capitis/longus colli muscles
G. erector spinae muscle
H. scalene muscles
I. external jugular vein
J. common carotid artery
K. submandibular gland

L. hyoid bone
M. mandible

Exercise 4-11: Labeling

A. hyoid bone
B. pharynx
C. anterior jugular vein
D. common carotid artery
E. vertebral artery
F. erector spinae muscle
G. anterior, middle, posterior scalene muscles
H. internal jugular vein
I. external jugular vein
J. SCM
K. submandibular gland
L. sternohyoid/sternothyroid muscles
M. platysma

Exercise 4-12: Labeling

A. pharynx
B. thyroid cartilage
C. anterior jugular vein
D. common carotid artery
E. internal jugular vein
F. vertebral artery
G. scalene muscles
H. erector spinae muscle
I. longus capitis/longus colli muscles
J. external jugular vein
K. SCM
L. sternohyoid/sternothyroid muscles
M. platysma

Exercise 4-13: Labeling

A. sternohyoid/sternothyroid muscle
B. SCM
C. internal jugular vein
D. longus capitis/longus colli muscle
E. scalene muscles
F. erector spinae muscle
G. vertebral artery
H. external jugular vein
I. common carotid artery
J. arytenoid

K. thyroid cartilage
L. pharynx

Exercise 4-14: Labeling

A. sternohyoid/sternothyroid muscle
B. pharynx
C. SCM
D. cricoid cartilage
E. internal jugular vein
F. vertebral artery
G. scalene muscles
H. erector spinae muscle
I. longus capitis/longus colli
J. external jugular vein
K. common carotid artery
L. thyroid gland
M. thyroid cartilage
N. platysma

Exercise 4-15: Labeling

A. sternohyoid/sternothyroid muscles
B. thyroid cartilage
C. cricoid cartilage
D. common carotid artery
E. longus capitis/longus colli muscles
F. vertebral artery
G. scalene muscles
H. erector spinae muscle
I. external jugular vein
J. internal jugular vein
K. thyroid gland
L. SCM
M. anterior jugular vein
N. platysma
O. pharynx

Exercise 4-16: Labeling

A. pharynx
B. sternohyoid/sternothyroid muscle
C. thyroid cartilage
D. thyroid gland
E. SCM
F. internal jugular vein
G. longus capitis/longus colli muscles
H. scalene muscles
I. erector spinae muscle

J. vertebral artery
K. external jugular vein
L. common carotid artery
M. thyroid gland
N. cricoid cartilage
O. anterior jugular vein
P. platysma

Exercise 4-17: Labeling

A. sternohyoid/sternothyroid muscles
B. cricoid cartilage
C. SCM
D. pharynx
E. internal jugular vein
F. longus colli
G. erector spinae muscle
H. common carotid artery
I. thyroid gland
J. anterior jugular vein
K. platysma

Exercise 4-18: Labeling

A. sternohyoid/sternothyroid muscle
B. pharynx
C. thyroid gland
D. internal jugular vein
E. longus colli muscle
F. anterior scalene muscle
G. middle and posterior scalene muscles
H. erector spinae muscle
I. external jugular vein
J. common carotid artery
K. SCM
L. cricoid cartilage
M. anterior jugular vein

Exercise 4-19: Labeling

A. sternohyoid/sternothyroid muscles
B. tracheal cartilage
C. trachea
D. internal jugular vein
E. longus colli muscle
F. anterior scalene muscle
G. middle/posterior scalene muscles
H. erector spinae muscle
I. esophagus

J. common carotid artery
K. thyroid gland
L. SCM
M. anterior jugular vein

Exercise 4-20: Labeling

A. pulmonary trunk
B. left pulmonary artery
C. descending aorta
D. right pulmonary artery
E. ascending aorta

Exercise 4-21: Labeling

A. left pulmonary artery
B. descending aorta
C. ascending aorta

Exercise 4-22: Labeling

A. left pulmonary artery
B. descending aorta
C. ascending aorta

Exercise 4-23: Labeling

A. descending aorta
B. ascending aorta

Exercise 4-24: Labeling

A. descending aorta
B. ascending aorta

Exercise 4-25: Labeling

A. arch of the aorta

Exercise 4-26: Labeling

A. arch of the aorta

Exercise 4-27: Labeling

A. arch of the aorta

Exercise 4-28: Labeling

A. arch of the aorta
B. right brachiocephalic artery

Exercise 4-29: Labeling

A. left common carotid artery
B. left subclavian artery
C. right brachiocephalic artery

Exercise 4-30: Labeling

A. left common carotid artery
B. left subclavian artery
C. right brachiocephalic artery

Exercise 4-31: Labeling

A. left common carotid artery
B. left subclavian artery
C. right brachiocephalic artery

Exercise 4-32: Labeling

A. left common carotid artery
B. left subclavian artery
C. right brachiocephalic artery

Exercise 4-33: Labeling

A. left common carotid artery
B. left subclavian artery
C. right brachiocephalic artery

Exercise 4-34: Labeling

A. left common carotid artery
B. left subclavian artery
C. bifurcation of right
   brachiocephalic artery

Exercise 4-35: Labeling

A. left common carotid artery
B. left subclavian artery
C. right subclavian artery
D. right common carotid artery

Exercise 4-36: Labeling

A. left common carotid artery
B. left subclavian artery
C. right subclavian artery
D. right common carotid artery

Exercise 4-37: Labeling

A. left common carotid artery
B. left subclavian artery
C. right subclavian artery
D. right common carotid artery

Exercise 4-38: Labeling

A. left common carotid artery
B. left subclavian artery
C. right subclavian artery
D. right common carotid artery

Exercise 4-39: Labeling

A. left common carotid artery
B. left subclavian artery
C. right subclavian artery
D. right common carotid artery

Exercise 4-40: Labeling

A. left common carotid artery
B. left subclavian artery
C. left vertebral artery
D. right subclavian artery
E. right common carotid artery

Exercise 4-41: Labeling

A. left common carotid artery
B. left vertebral artery
C. right vertebral artery
D. right common carotid artery

Exercise 4-42: Labeling

A. left common carotid artery
B. left vertebral artery
C. right vertebral artery
D. right common carotid artery

Exercise 4-43: Labeling

A. left common carotid artery
B. left vertebral artery
C. right vertebral artery
D. right common carotid artery

Exercise 4-44: Labeling

A. left common carotid artery
B. left vertebral artery
C. right vertebral artery
D. right common carotid artery

Exercise 4-45: Labeling

A. left common carotid artery
B. left vertebral artery
C. right vertebral artery
D. right common carotid artery

Exercise 4-46: Labeling

A. left common carotid artery
B. left vertebral artery
C. right vertebral artery
D. right common carotid artery

Exercise 4-47: Labeling

A. left common carotid artery
B. left vertebral artery
C. right vertebral artery
D. right common carotid artery

Exercise 4-48: Labeling

A. left common carotid artery
B. left vertebral artery
C. right vertebral artery
D. right common carotid artery

Exercise 4-49: Labeling

A. middle cerebral artery
B. posterior cerebral artery
C. basilar artery
D. vertebral artery
E. left subclavian artery
F. arch of aorta
G. left common carotid artery
H. right brachiocephalic artery
I. right common carotid artery
J. right subclavian artery
K. external carotid artery
L. internal carotid artery
M. anterior cerebral artery

Exercise 4-50: Labeling

A. anterior communicating artery
B. left posterior cerebral artery
C. basilar artery
D. left internal carotid artery
E. left external carotid artery
F. left vertebral artery
G. left subclavian artery
H. left common carotid artery
I. arch of aorta
J. right brachiocephalic artery
K. right subclavian artery
L. right vertebral artery
M. right internal carotid artery
N. right middle cerebral artery
O. right anterior cerebral artery

Exercise 4-51: Labeling

A. anterior communicating artery
B. internal carotid artery
C. middle cerebral artery
D. posterior communicating artery
E. posterior cerebral artery
F. basilar artery
G. posterior cerebral artery
H. middle cerebral artery
I. internal carotid artery
J. anterior cerebral artery

CHAPTER 5: THORAX

Exercise 5-1: Labeling

A. right ventricle
B. left ventricle
C. left atrium
D. right atrium

Exercise 5-2: Matching

1. b
2. c
3. d
4. a

Exercise 5-3: Term Identification

1. cardiac notch
2. xiphoid or ensiform process
3. foramen ovale
4. sternal angle
5. visceral

Exercise 5-4: Identification

1. SVC
2. IVC
3. pulmonary trunk
4. aorta

Exercise 5-5: Term Identification

1. suprasternal notch
2. bicuspid valve
3. epicardium
4. ensiform process

Exercise 5-6: Labeling

A. left common carotid artery
B. left subclavian artery
C. aortic arch
D. aorta
E. descending aorta
F. left pulmonary artery
G. left pulmonary veins
H. left atrium
I. aortic semilunar valve
J. bicuspid (mitral) valve
K. left ventricle
L. Septum
M. inferior vena cava
N. right ventricle

O. tricuspid valve
P. right atrium
Q. pulmonary semilunar valve
R. right pulmonary veins
S. pulmonary trunk
T. right pulmonary artery
U. superior vena cava
V. ascending aorta
W. brachiocephalic artery

Exercise 5-7: Abbreviations

1. Inferior Vena Cava
2. Sternoclavicular
3. Superior Vena Cava

Exercise 5-8: Labeling

A. myocardium
B. endocardium
C. serous pericardium (epicardium)
D. space
E. serous pericardium (parietal layer)
F. fibrous pericardium

Exercise 5-9: Completion

(Terms listed in the order they appear.)
deoxygenated
right atrium
SVC
IVC
coronary sinus
tricuspid valve
right ventricle
pulmonary trunk
pulmonary semilunar valve
pulmonary circulatory system
pulmonary trunk
pulmonary arteries
lungs
capillaries
alveoli
pulmonary veins
left atrium
oxygenated
bicuspid valve
mitral valve
left ventricle
aorta
aortic semilunar valve
systemic circulatory system

Exercise 5-10: Sorting

1. D
2. C
3. B
4. A
5. E

Exercise 5-11: Identification

1. C
2. C
3. B
4. A
5. D
6. C
7. C
8. D
9. A
10. C

Exercise 5-12: Labeling

A. suprasternal/jugular notch
B. thymus
C. trachea
D. left subclavian artery
E. left common carotid artery
F. levator scapulae muscle
G. trapezius muscle
H. erector spinae muscle
I. apex of right lung
J. esophagus
K. clavicle
L. sternoclavicular joint
M. manubrium

Exercise 5-13: Labeling

A. pectoralis major
B. pectoralis minor
C. left brachiocephalic (innominate) vein
D. left subclavian artery
E. left common carotid artery
F. latissimus dorsi muscle
G. trachea
H. tubercle of rib
I. levator scapulae muscle
J. trapezius muscle
K. rhomboid muscle
L. head of rib
M. serratus anterior muscle

N. esophagus
O. right subclavian artery
P. right brachiocephalic vein
Q. right common carotid artery

Exercise 5-14: Labeling

A. pectoralis major muscle
B. pectoralis minor muscle
C. left brachiocephalic vein
D. left subclavian artery
E. left common carotid artery
F. esophagus
G. erector spinae muscle
H. trapezius muscle
I. intercostal muscle
J. trachea
K. serratus anterior muscle
L. right subclavian artery
M. right brachiocephalic vein
N. right common carotid artery

Exercise 5-15: Labeling

A. pectoralis major muscle
B. pectoralis minor muscle
C. left brachiocephalic vein
D. left common carotid artery
E. latissimus dorsi muscle
F. left subclavian artery
G. trachea
H. levator scapulae muscle
I. trapezius muscle
J. rhomboid muscle
K. erector spinae muscle
L. esophagus
M. serratus anterior muscle
N. right subclavian artery
O. right brachiocephalic vein
P. right common carotid artery

Exercise 5-16: Labeling

A. pectoralis major muscle
B. margin of mediastinum
C. pectoralis minor muscle
D. left brachiocephalic vein
E. left common carotid artery
F. serratus anterior muscle
G. left subclavian artery
H. tubercle of rib
I. erector spinae muscle
J. trapezius muscle

K. head of rib
L. esophagus
M. trachea
N. right brachiocephalic vein
O. right brachiocephalic artery

Exercise 5-17: Labeling

A. pectoralis major muscle
B. pectoralis minor muscle
C. left brachiocephalic vein
D. serratus anterior muscle
E. portion of arch of aorta
F. latissimus dorsi muscle
G. esophagus
H. erector spinae muscle
I. trapezius muscle
J. rhomboid muscle
K. intercostal muscle
L. trachea
M. right brachiocephalic vein
N. right brachiocehalic artery

Exercise 5-18: Labeling

A. body of sternum
B. intercostal muscle
C. arch of aorta
D. latissimus dorsi muscle
E. esophagus
F. erector spinae muscle
G. trapezius muscle
H. rhomboid muscle
I. trachea
J. serratus anterior muscle
K. formation of superior vena cava
L. pectoralis minor muscle
M. pectoralis major muscle

Exercise 5-19: Labeling

A. ascending aorta
B. serratus anterior muscle
C. latissimus dorsi muscle
D. descending aorta
E. rhomboid muscle
F. trapezius muscle
G. erector spinae muscle
H. esophagus
I. trachea
J. superior vena cava
K. pectoralis minor muscle
L. pectoralis major muscle

Exercise 5-20: Labeling

A. ascending aorta
B. intercostal muscle
C. arch of aorta
D. latissimus dorsi muscle
E. thoracic descending aorta
F. rhomboid major muscle
G. trapezius muscle
H. erector spinae muscle
I. esophagus
J. trachea
K. serratus anterior muscle
L. superior vena cava
M. pectoralis minor muscle
N. pectoralis major muscle

Exercise 5-21: Labeling

A. ascending aorta
B. pulmonary trunk
C. latissimus dorsi muscle
D. descending aorta
E. trapezius muscle
F. erector spinae muscle
G. esophagus
H. azygos arch
I. serratus anterior muscle
J. trachea
K. superior vena cava
L. pectoralis major muscle

Exercise 5-22: Labeling

A. ascending aorta
B. pulmonary trunk
C. serratus anterior muscle
D. left primary bronchus
E. left pulmonary artery
F. latissimus dorsi muscle
G. descending aorta
H. esophagus
I. erector spinae muscle
J. trapezius muscle
K. azygos vein
L. carina
M. right primary bronchus
N. hilum
O. right pulmonary artery
P. superior vena cava
Q. pectoralis major muscle

Exercise 5-23: Labeling

A. pectoralis major muscle
B. ascending aorta

C. pulmonary trunk
D. serratus anterior muscle
E. left pulmonary artery
F. latissimus dorsi muscle
G. left primary bronchus
H. descending aorta
I. rhomboid major muscle
J. trapezius muscle
K. azygos vein
L. esophagus
M. right primary bronchus
N. hilum
O. intercostal muscle
P. right pulmonary artery
Q. superior vena cava

Exercise 5-24: Labeling

A. pulmonary trunk
B. left pulmonary artery
C. serratus anterior muscle
D. left primary bronchus
E. latissimus dorsi muscle
F. esophagus
G. descending aorta
H. trapezius muscle
I. erector spinae muscle
J. azygos vein
K. right primary bronchus
L. hilum
M. right pulmonary artery
N. intercostal muscle
O. superior vena cava
P. ascending aorta
Q. pectoralis major
   muscle

Exercise 5-25: Labeling

A. pectoralis major muscle
B. pulmonary trunk
C. serratus anterior muscle
D. left secondary bronchi
E. descending aorta
F. rhomboid major muscle
G. azygos vein
H. esophagus
I. superior vena cava
J. ascending aorta

Exercise 5-26: Labeling

A. intercostal muscle
B. left atrium

C. left pulmonary vein
D. descending aorta
E. erector spinae muscle
F. rhomboid major muscle
G. azygos vein
H. esophagus
I. right pulmonary vein
J. superior vena cava
K. serratus anterior muscle
L. ascending aorta
M. right atrium

Exercise 5-27: Labeling

A. right ventricle
B. ascending aorta
C. left ventricle
D. left atrium
E. latissimus dorsi muscle
F. left pulmonary vein
G. descending aorta
H. trapezius muscle
I. azygos vein
J. esophagus
K. right pulmonary vein
L. superior vena cava
M. serratus anterior muscle
N. right atrium

Exercise 5-28: Labeling

A. right ventricle
B. interventricular septum
C. left ventricle
D. intercostal muscle
E. bicuspid/mitral valve
F. latissimus dorsi
   muscle
G. descending aorta
H. trapezius muscle
I. erector spinae
   muscle
J. azygos vein
K. esophagus
L. left atrium
M. serratus anterior muscle
N. interatrial septum
O. ascending aorta
P. right atrium

Exercise 5-29: Labeling

A. right ventricle
B. left ventricle
C. latissimus dorsi muscle

D. descending aorta
E. azygos vein
F. esophagus
G. left atrium
H. serratus anterior muscle
I. interatrial septum
J. ascending aorta
K. right atrium
L. tricuspid valve

Exercise 5-30: Labeling

A. right ventricle
B. left ventricle
C. left atrium
D. descending aorta
E. trapezius muscle
F. azygos vein
G. esophagus
H. intercostal muscle
I. serratus anterior muscle
J. right atrium

Exercise 5-31: Labeling

A. right ventricle
B. left ventricle
C. descending aorta
D. erector spinae muscle
E. azygos vein
F. esophagus
G. left atrium
H. serratus anterior muscle
I. pericardium

Exercise 5-32: Labeling

A. right ventricle
B. interventricular septum
C. left ventricle
D. descending aorta
E. intercostal muscle
F. erector spinae muscle
G. azygos vein
H. esophagus
I. left atrium
J. serratus anterior muscle
K. xiphoid process of sternum

Exercise 5-33: Labeling

A. right ventricle
B. interventricular septum
C. serratus anterior muscle

D. left ventricle
E. descending aorta
F. azygos vein
G. esophagus
H. left atrium
I. inferior vena cava

Exercise 5-34: Labeling

A. right ventricle
B. left ventricle
C. descending aorta
D. erector spinae muscle
E. azygos vein
F. esophagus
G. IVC
H. serratus anterior muscle
I. diaphragm
J. intercostal muscle
K. liver

CHAPTER 6: ABDOMEN

Exercise 6-1: Identification

1. caval hiatus
2. esophageal hiatus
3. aortic hiatus

Exercise 6-2: Identification

1. celiac axis or trunk
2. SMA
3. right/left renal arteries
4. IMA

Exercise 6-3: Identification

1. splenic artery
2. left gastric artery
3. common hepatic artery

Exercise 6-4: Identification

1. splenic vein
2. SMV

Exercise 6-5: Matching

1. i
2. a
3. e
4. j
5. c
6. f

7. b
8. h
9. d
10. g

Exercise 6-6: Identification

1. right
2. left
3. caudate
4. quadrate

Exercise 6-7: Matching

1. a
2. b
3. c
4. c
5. b
6. c

Exercise 6-8: Labeling

A. hepatic portal vein
B. inferior vena cava
C. common bile duct
D. cystic duct
E. right lobe
F. common hepatic duct
G. gallbladder
H. quadrate lobe
I. longitudinal fissure
J. falciform ligament
K. ligamentum teres
L. right hepatic duct
M. left hepatic duct
N. right hepatic artery
O. left hepatic artery
P. left lobe
Q. ligementum venosum
R. caudate lobe
S. round ligament
T. umbilical notch

Exercise 6-9: Matching

1. b
2. c
3. a

Exercise 6-10: Identification

1. A
2. B

3. A
4. A

Exercise 6-11: Labeling

A. anterior pararenal compartment
B. peritoneum
C. stomach
D. spleen
E. pancreas
F. descending colon
G. duodenum
H. left kidney
I. posterior pararenal compartment
J. aorta
K. perirenal space
L. right kidney
M. ascending colon
N. inferior vena cava
O. liver

Exercise 6-12: Identification

1. C
2. C
3. B
4. C
5. B
6. A
7. C
8. A
9. A
10. B
11. A
12. A
13. C

Exercise 6-13: Identification

1. A
2. B
3. A
4. B
5. B
6. A
7. B

Exercise 6-14: Labeling

A. pericardium
B. interventricular septum
C. left ventricle
D. esophagus

E. descending aorta
F. hemiazygos vein
G. lung
H. azygos vein
I. inferior vena cava
J. right hepatic vein
K. right lobe of liver
L. middle hepatic vein
M. right ventricle

Exercise 6-15: Labeling

A. interventricular septum
B. left ventricle
C. descending aorta
D. hemiazygos vein
E. spleen
F. lung
G. azygos vein
H. IVC
I. right hepatic vein
J. right lobe of liver
K. middle hepatic vein
L. right ventricle

Exercise 6-16: Labeling

A. lung
B. esophagus
C. descending aorta
D. hemiazygos vein
E. spleen
F. azygos vein
G. IVC
H. right lobe of liver

Exercise 6-17: Labeling

A. lung
B. fundus of stomach
C. descending aorta
D. spleen
E. right crus of diaphragm
F. right adrenal
G. IVC
H. right lobe of liver
I. esophagus
J. left lobe of liver

Exercise 6-18: Labeling

A. left lobe of liver
B. lung
C. esophagogastric junction
D. stomach

E. descending aorta
F. spleen
G. left crus of diaphragm
H. right crus of diaphragm
I. right kidney
J. right adrenal
K. IVC
L. caudate lobe of liver
M. right lobe of liver

Exercise 6-19: Labeling

A. left lobe of liver
B. greater curvature of stomach
C. stomach
D. lesser curvature of stomach
E. descending aorta
F. left crus of diaphragm
G. spleen
H. right crus of diaphragm
I. right kidney
J. right adrenal
K. IVC
L. right lobe of liver
M. caudate lobe of liver
N. ligamentum venosum

Exercise 6-20: Labeling

A. rectus abdominis muscle
B. stomach
C. splenic artery
D. left crus of diaphragm
E. spleen
F. left adrenal
G. erector spinae muscle
H. right kidney
I. right lobe of liver
J. right adrenal
K. caudate lobe of liver
L. ligamentum venosum
M. left lobe of liver
N. linea alba

Exercise 6-21: Labeling

A. linea alba
B. rectus abdominis muscle
C. stomach
D. spleen
E. splenic artery
F. left adrenal
G. left crus of diahragm
H. left kidney

I. erector spinae muscle
J. right kidney
K. right crus of diaphragm
L. IVC
M. right lobe of liver
N. caudate lobe of liver
O. ligamentum venosum
P. left lobe of liver

Exercise 6-22: Labeling

A. linea alba
B. left lobe of liver
C. stomach
D. descending aorta
E. splenic artery
F. left adrenal
G. spleen
H. left kidney
I. erector spinae muscle
J. cortex of kidney
K. medulla of kidney
L. right kidney
M. hilum of kidney
N. IVC
O. right lobe of liver
P. falciform ligament
Q. rectus abdominis muscle

Exercise 6-23: Labeling

A. stomach
B. left gastric artery
C. spleen
D. splenic vein
E. tail of pancreas
F. descending aorta
G. left kidney
H. IVC
I. right lobe of liver
J. celiac axis
K. portal vein
L. gallbladder
M. common hepatic artery
N. falciform ligament
O. left lobe of liver

Exercise 6-24: Labeling

A. rectus abdominis muscle
B. left lobe of liver
C. stomach
D. splenic flexure
E. body of pancreas

F. splenic vein
G. spleen
H. erector spinae muscle
I. right kidney
J. right ureter
K. descending aorta
L. superior mesenteric artery
M. portal vein
N. gallbladder
O. quadrate lobe of liver
P. falciform ligament

Exercise 6-25: Labeling

A. left lobe of liver
B. body of pancreas
C. splenic flexure
D. splenic vein
E. tail of pancreas
F. superior mesenteric artery
G. IVC
H. medulla of kidney
I. cortex of kidney
J. right renal vein
K. duodenum
L. superior mesenteric vein
M. head of pancreas
N. gallbladder
O. quadrate lobe of liver
P. ligamentum teres

Exercise 6-26: Labeling

A. head of pancreas
B. body of pancreas
C. splenic flexure
D. anterior pararenal space
E. left renal vein
F. spleen
G. psoas muscle
H. posterior pararenal space
I. descending aorta
J. right renal vein
K. IVC
L. duodenum
M. SMA
N. SMV
O. gallbladder
P. quadrate lobe of liver
Q. ligamentum teres

Exercise 6-27: Labeling

A. rectus abdominis muscle
B. left lobe of liver

C. distal stomach
D. ligamentum teres
E. gallbladder
F. IVC
G. spleen
H. descending colon
I. psoas muscle
J. descending aorta
K. right renal artery
L. duodenum
M. right lobe of liver
N. SMA
O. SMV
P. pylorus
Q. quadrate lobe of liver

Exercise 6-28: Labeling

A. linea alba
B. stomach
C. jejunum
D. spleen
E. descending colon
F. left ureter
G. descending aorta
H. IVC
I. erector spinae muscle
J. psoas muscle
K. SMA
L. right lobe of liver
M. SMV
N. gallbladder
O. pylorus
P. quadrate lobe of liver
Q. left lobe of liver

Exercise 6-29: Labeling

A. jejunum
B. spleen
C. descending aorta
D. descending colon
E. left ureter
F. psoas muscle
G. left kidney
H. erector spinae muscle
I. right lobe of liver
J. IVC
K. hepatic flexure
L. SMA
M. SMV
N. gallbladder
O. falciform ligament
P. left lobe of liver

Exercise 6-30: Labeling

A. linea alba
B. rectus abdominis
C. stomach
D. spleen
E. descending colon
F. left ureter
G. left kidney
H. psoas muscle
I. IVC
J. right kidney
K. right lobe of liver
L. SMA
M. SMV
N. hepatic flexure
O. pylorus
P. left lobe of liver

Exercise 6-31: Labeling

A. rectus abdominis muscle
B. stomach
C. spleen
D. SMA
E. descending aorta
F. descending colon
G. psoas muscle
H. left kidney
I. erector spinae muscle
J. right kidney
K. right lobe of liver
L. IVC
M. SMV
N. hepatic flexure
O. left lobe of liver
P. linea alba

Exercise 6-32: Labeling

A. external oblique muscle
B. internal oblique muscle
C. transversus abdominis muscle
D. spleen
E. descending aorta
F. erector spinae muscle
G. psoas muscle
H. IVC
I. liver
J. hepatic flexure

Exercise 6-33: Labeling

A. linea alba
B. external oblique muscle
C. internal oblique muscle
D. transversus abdominis muscle
E. spleen
F. left kidney
G. quadratus lumborum muscle
H. erector spinae muscle
I. psoas muscle
J. liver
K. IVC
L. descending aorta
M. transverse colon
N. rectus abdominis muscle

Exercise 6-34: Labeling

A. external oblique muscle
B. internal oblique muscle
C. transversus abdominis muscle
D. spleen
E. descending aorta
F. erector spinae muscle
G. quadratus lumborum muscle
H. psoas muscle
I. IVC
J. transverse colon
K. rectus abdominis muscle
L. linea alba

Exercise 6-35: Labeling

A. linea alba
B. external oblique muscle
C. internal oblique muscle
D. transversus abdominis muscle
E. descending aorta
F. quadratus lumborum muscle
G. erector spinae muscle
H. psoas muscle
I. IVC
J. rectus abdominis muscle

Exercise 6-36: Labeling

A. umbilicus
B. linea alba
C. external oblique muscle
D. internal oblique muscle
E. transversus abdominis muscle
F. left common iliac artery
G. quadratus lumborum muscle
H. erector spinae muscle
I. psoas muscle
J. IVC

K. right common iliac artery
L. rectus abdominis muscle

Exercise 6-37

A. linea alba
B. rectus abdominis muscle
C. left common iliac artery
D. psoas muscle
E. iliac crest
F. erector spinae muscle
G. IVC
H. right common iliac artery
I. transversus abdominis muscle
J. internal oblique muscle
K. external oblique muscle

Exercise 6-38: Labeling

A. left ventricle of heart
B. descending aorta
C. lung
D. erector spinae muscle
E. liver
F. IVC
G. right ventricle of heart

Exercise 6-39: Labeling

A. linea alba
B. left ventricle of heart
C. esophagus
D. descending aorta
E. erector spinae muscle
F. liver
G. IVC
H. right ventricle of heart
I. rectus abdominis muscle

Exercise 6-40: Labeling

A. linea alba
B. left ventricle of heart
C. esophagus
D. descending aorta
E. erector spinae muscle
F. liver
G. IVC
H. right ventricle of heart
I. rectus abdominis muscle

Exercise 6-41: Labeling

A. linea alba
B. left lobe of liver

C. esophagus
D. descending aorta
E. fundus of stomach
F. erector spinae muscle
G. right lobe of liver
H. right hepatic vein
I. IVC
J. middle hepatic vein
K. left hepatic vein
L. rectus abdominis muscle

Exercise 6-42: Labeling

A. linea alba
B. left lobe of liver
C. esophagus
D. stomach
E. descending aorta
F. erector spinae muscle
G. right lobe of liver
H. right hepatic vein
I. IVC
J. middle hepatic vein
K. left hepatic vein
L. rectus abdominis muscle

Exercise 6-43: Labeling

A. linea alba
B. left lobe of liver
C. esophagus
D. stomach
E. descending aorta
F. erector spinae muscle
G. right lobe of liver
H. right hepatic vein
I. IVC
J. middle hepatic vein
K. left hepatic vein
L. rectus abodminis muscle

Exercise 6-44: Labeling

A. linea alba
B. left lobe of liver
C. ligamentum venosum
D. esophagogastric junction
E. descending aorta
F. spleen
G. erector spinae muscle
H. right lobe of liver
I. IVC
J. caudate lobe of liver
K. rectus abdominis muscle

Exercise 6-45: Labeling

A. linea alba
B. left lobe of liver
C. body of stomach
D. descending aorta
E. spleen
F. left crus of diaphragm
G. erector spinae muscle
H. right lobe of liver
I. IVC
J. caudate lobe of liver
K. rectus abdominis muscle

Exercise 6-46: Labeling

A. rectus abdominis muscle
B. left lobe of liver
C. stomach
D. descending aorta
E. spleen
F. erector spinae muscle
G. right lobe of liver
H. IVC
I. caudate lobe of liver
J. linea alba

Exercise 6-47: Labeling

A. rectus abdominis mucle
B. left lobe of liver
C. ligamentum venosum
D. stomach
E. descending aorta
F. left adrenal
G. spleen
H. left kidney
I. erector spinae muscle
J. right lobe of liver
K. right crus of diaphragm
L. IVC
M. caudate lobe of liver
N. portal vein
O. linea alba

Exercise 6-48: Labeling

A. rectus abdominis muscle
B. left lobe of liver
C. stomach
D. descending aorta
E. spleen
F. left kidney
G. erector spinae muscle

H. right crus of diaphragm
I. IVC
J. caudate lobe of liver
K. portal vein
L. linea alba

Exercise 6-49: Labeling

A. rectus abdominis muscle
B. stomach
C. descending aorta
D. left crus of diaphragm
E. spleen
F. left kidney
G. erector spinae muscle
H. right lobe of liver
I. IVC
J. falciform ligament
K. linea alba

Exercise 6-50: Labeling

A. rectus abdominis muscle
B. left lobe of liver
C. stomach
D. descending aorta
E. spleen
F. left kidney
G. erector spinae muscle
H. right lobe of liver
I. right adrenal
J. right crus of diaphragm
K. IVC
L. falciform ligament
M. linea alba

Exercise 6-51: Labeling

A. body of pancreas
B. descending aorta
C. spleen
D. left kidney
E. erector spinae muscle
F. right kidney
G. right lobe of liver
H. falciform ligament
I. left lobe of liver

Exercise 6-52: Labeling

A. left lobe of liver
B. left renal vein
C. descending aorta
D. spleen
E. left kidney

F. cortex of kidney
G. erector spinae muscle
H. right kidney
I. IVC
J. gallbladder
K. falciform ligament

Exercise 6-53: Labeling

A. left kidney
B. erector spinae muscle
C. right kidney
D. right lobe of liver
E. gallbladder

Exercise 6-54: Labeling

A. left kidney
B. psoas muscle
C. erector spinae muscle
D. right kidney
E. right lobe of liver
F. gallbladder

Exercise 6-55: Labeling

A. psoas muscle
B. left kidney
C. erector spinae muscle
D. right kidney
E. liver
F. gallbladder

Exercise 6-56: Labeling

A. left kidney
B. psoas muscle
C. erector spinae muscle
D. right kidney
E. liver
F. gallbladder

Exercise 6-57: Labeling

A. splenic flexure
B. psoas muscle
C. left kidney
D. quadratus lumborum muscle
E. erector spinae muscle
F. right kidney
G. liver
H. gallbladder

Exercise 6-58: Labeling

A. descending colon
B. psoas muscle

C. left kidney
D. quadratus lumborum muscle
E. erector spinae muscle
F. cortex right kidney
G. liver

Exercise 6-59: Labeling

A. psoas muscle
B. left kidney
C. erector spinae muscle
D. quadratus lumborum muscle
E. right kidney
F. liver
G. hepatic flexure

Exercise 6-60: Labeling

A. psoas muscle
B. left kidney
C. erector spinae muscle
D. quadratus lumborum muscle
E. right kidney
F. liver

Exercise 6-61: Labeling

A. internal oblique muscle
B. transversus abdominis muscle
C. external oblique muscle
D. psoas muscle
E. left kidney
F. erector spinae muscle
G. quadratus lumborum muscle
H. right kidney

Exercise 6-62: Labeling

A. psoas muscle
B. left kidney
C. erector spinae muscle
D. quadratus lumborum muscle
E. right kidney
F. lateral muscles

Exercise 6-63: Labeling

A. transversus abdominis muscle
B. internal oblique muscle
C. external oblique muscle
D. psoas muscle
E. left kidney
F. erector spinae muscle
G. quadratus lumborum muscle
H. right kidney

Exercise 6-64: Labeling

A. psoas muscle
B. quadratus lumborum muscle
C. erector spinae muscle
D. right kidney
E. transversus abdominis muscle
F. internal oblique muscle
G. external oblique muscle

Exercise 6-65: Labeling

A. psoas muscle
B. quadratus lumborum muscle
C. erector spinae muscle
D. right kidney
E. transversus abdominis muscle
F. internal oblique muscle
G. external oblique muscle

Exercise 6-66: Labeling

A. external oblique muscle
B. internal oblique muscle
C. transversus abdominis muscle
D. erector spinae muscle
E. quadratus lumborum muscle
F. right kidney
G. psoas muscle
H. ascending colon

Exercise 6-67: Labeling

A. external oblique muscle
B. internal oblique muscle
C. transversus abdominis muscle
D. erector spinae muscle
E. quadratus lumborum muscle
F. right kidney
G. psoas muscle

Exercise 6-68: Labeling

A. lateral muscles
B. erector spinae muscle
C. quadratus lumborum muscle
D. psoas muscle

Exercise 6-69: Labeling

A. erector spinae muscle

Exercise 6-70: Labeling

A. intercostal muscle
B. erector spinae muscle

Exercise 6-71: Labeling

A. intercostal muscle
B. erector spinae muscle
C. lung

Exercise 6-72: Labeling

A. erector spinae muscle
B. liver
C. lung

Exercise 6-73: Labeling

A. spleen
B. left kidney
C. erector spinae muscle
D. liver
E. lung

Exercise 6-74: Labeling

A. spleen
B. left kidney
C. erector spinae muscle
D. quadratus lumborum muscle
E. right kidney
F. spinal canal
G. liver
H. lung

Exercise 6-75: Labeling

A. spleen
B. left kidney
C. spinal canal
D. quadratus lumborum muscle
E. right kidney
F. liver
G. diaphragm
H. lung

Exercise 6-76: Labeling

A. left hemidiaphragm
B. spleen
C. left kidney
D. quadratus lumborum muscle
E. right kidney
F. liver
G. right hemidiaphragm
H. right lung

Exercise 6-77: Labeling

A. spleen
B. cortex left kidney

C. hilum of kidney
D. psoas muscle
E. spinal canal
F. right kidney
G. liver
H. diaphragm
I. lung

Exercise 6-78: Labeling

A. spleen
B. left kidney
C. psoas muscle
D. right kidney
E. liver
F. diaphragm
G. lung

Exercise 6-79: Labeling

A. thoracic descending aorta
B. spleen
C. left kidney
D. psoas muscle
E. right kidney
F. liver
G. hepatic vein
H. IVC

Exercise 6-80: Labeling

A. descending aorta
B. spleen
C. left kidney
D. psoas muscle
E. right kidney
F. right adrenal
G. liver
H. IVC

Exercise 6-81: Labeling

A. stomach
B. descending aorta
C. spleen
D. pancreas
E. psoas muscle
F. right kidney
G. liver
H. IVC

Exercise 6-82: Labeling

A. stomach
B. pancreas
C. abdominal descending aorta

D. spleen
E. descending colon
F. lateral muscles
G. ascending colon
H. IVC
I. liver
J. diaphragm

Exercise 6-83: Labeling

A. stomach
B. esophagogastric junction
C. pancreas
D. descending colon
E. lateral muscle
F. ascending colon
G. gallbladder
H. liver
I. diaphragm

Exercise 6-84: Labeling

A. left lobe of liver
B. stomach
C. pancreas
D. lateral muscles
E. descending colon
F. ascending colon
G. SMV
H. gallbladder
I. right lobe of liver
J. portal vein

Exercise 6-85: Labeling

A. left lobe of liver
B. stomach
C. pancreas
D. descending colon
E. lateral muscles
F. ascending colon
G. gallbladder
H. SMV
I. right lobe of liver

Exercise 6-86: Labeling

A. heart
B. left lobe of liver
C. stomach
D. splenic flexure
E. lateral muscles
F. transverse colon
G. hepatic flexure
H. right lobe of liver
I. diaphragm

Exercise 6-87: Labeling

A. heart
B. left lobe of liver
C. stomach
D. splenic flexure
E. transverse colon
F. transverse colon
G. hepatic flexure
H. right lobe of liver
I. diaphragm

Exercise 6-88: Labeling

A. heart
B. stomach
C. greater curvature of stomach
D. pylorus
E. transverse colon
F. right lobe of liver
G. diaphragm

Exercise 6-89: Labeling

A. heart
B. left lobe of liver
C. stomach
D. lesser curvature
E. greater curvature
F. right lobe of liver
G. diaphragm

Exercise 6-90: Labeling

A. heart
B. left lobe of liver
C. stomach
D. falciform ligament
E. right lobe of liver
F. diaphragm
G. lung

Exercise 6-91: Labeling

A. stomach
B. linea alba
C. rectus abdominis muscle
D. right lobe of liver
E. diaphragm
F. lung

Exercise 6-92: Labeling

A. stomach
B. linea alba
C. rectus abdominis muscle

D. liver
E. lung

Exercise 6-93: Labeling

A. sternum
B. rib
C. rectus abdominis muscle

CHAPTER 7: PELVIS

Exercise 7-1: Completion

(Terms listed in the order they appear.)
testis
testicles
epididymis
scrotum
ductus vas deferens
seminal vesicles
seminal vesicle duct
ejaculatory duct
prostatic urethra
prostate gland
prostate gland
prostate gland
bulbourethral glands
Cowper's glands

Exercise 7-2: Identification

1. fundus
2. body
3. cervix

Exercise 7-3: Matching

1. e
2. c
3. f
4. a
5. b
6. d

Exercise 7-4: Sorting

1. 2
2. 1
3. 3

Exercise 7-5: Matching

1. d
2. c

3. b
4. f
5. e
6. a

Exercise 7-6: Matching

1. e
2. c
3. h
4. a
5. i
6. b
7. j
8. d
9. f
10. g

Exercise 7-7: Labeling

A. urinary bladder
B. ductus vas deferens
C. prostate gland
D. prostatic urethra
E. urethra
F. epididymis
G. seminiferous tubules
H. testis
I. scrotum
J. bulbourethral gland
K. ejaculatory duct
L. seminal vesicle
M. rectum

Exercise 7-8: Labeling

A. uterine cavity
B. uterine tube
C. infundibulum
D. fimbriae
E. vagina
F. fornix
G. cervix of uterus
H. body of uterus
I. ovary
J. fundus of uterus

Exercise 7-9: Labeling

A. descending colon
B. external oblique muscle
C. internal oblique muscle
D. transversus abdominis muscle
E. left common iliac artery

F. left ureter
G. iliac crest
H. psoas muscle
I. IVC
J. right ureter
K. right common iliac artery
L. rectus abdominis muscle
M. linea alba

Exercise 7-10: Labeling

A. descending colon
B. left common iliac artery
C. lateral muscles
D. left ureter
E. left common iliac vein
F. iliacus muscle
G. psoas muscle
H. ilium
I. gluteal medius muscle
J. right common iliac vein
K. right ureter
L. right common iliac artery
M. ileum
N. cecum
O. rectus abdominis muscle
P. linea alba

Exercise 7-11: Labeling

A. descending colon
B. external oblique muscle
C. internal oblique muscle
D. transversus abdominis muscle
E. left common iliac artery
F. left common iliac vein
G. psoas muscle
H. iliacus muscle
I. gluteal maximus muscle
J. ilium
K. gluteal medius muscle
L. right common iliac vein
M. right common iliac artery
N. right ureter
O. rectus abdominis muscle
P. linea alba

Exercise 7-12: Labeling

A. descending colon
B. psoas muscle
C. left common iliac artery
D. left common iliac vein
E. iliacus muscle

F. SI joint
G. gluteal maximus muscle
H. erector spinae muscle
I. sacral promontory
J. gluteal medius muscle
K. right internal iliac vein
L. right external iliac vein
M. right common iliac artery
N. lateral muscles

Exercise 7-13: Labeling

A. left external iliac artery
B. left external iliac vein
C. left internal iliac artery
D. left internal iliac vein
E. gluteal minimus muscle
F. gluteal medius muscle
G. gluteal maximus muscle
H. sacrum
I. SI joint
J. iliacus muscle
K. psoas muscle
L. rectus abdominis muscle
M. linea alba

Exercise 7-14: Labeling

A. iliopsoas muscle
B. ilium
C. SI joint
D. sacrum
E. gluteal maximus muscle
F. gluteal medius muscle
G. gluteal minimus muscle
H. right external iliac vein
I. right external iliac artery

Exercise 7-15: Labeling

A. linea alba
B. iliopsoas muscle
C. left external iliac artery
D. left external iliac vein
E. gluteal minimus muscle
F. gluteal medius muscle
G. gluteal maximus muscle
H. sacrum
I. piriformis muscle
J. fundus of uterus
K. right internal iliac vein
L. right internal iliac artery
M. right external iliac artery and vein

N. bladder
O. rectus abdominis muscle

Exercise 7-16: Labeling

A. linea alba
B. left external iliac artery
C. left external iliac vein
D. iliopsoas muscle
E. ovary
F. uterus
G. gluteal maximus muscle
H. piriformis muscle
I. uterine cavity
J. right external iliac vein
K. right external iliac artery
L. sartorius muscle
M. rectus abdominis muscle

Exercise 7-17: Labeling

A. left external iliac artery
B. left external iliac vein
C. bladder
D. ovary
E. uterus
F. gluteal maximus muscle
G. right external iliac vein
H. right external iliac artery
I. iliopsoas muscle
J. tensor muscle
K. sartorius muscle

Exercise 7-18: Labeling

A. bladder
B. sartorius muscle
C. tensor muscle
D. left external iliac artery
E. left external iliac vein
F. uterus
G. coccyx
H. gluteal maximus muscle
I. acetabulum
J. head of femur
K. iliopsoas muscle
L. right external iliac vein
M. right external iliac artery

Exercise 7-19: Labeling

A. sartorius muscle
B. tensor muscle
C. rectus femoris muscle

D. bladder
E. head of femur
F. greater trochanter
G. cervix
H. ischial spine
I. coccyx
J. gluteal maximus muscle
K. rectum
L. ischium
M. superior pubic ramus
N. iliopsoas muscle
O. right external iliac vein
P. right external iliac artery

Exercise 7-20: Labeling

A. sartorius muscle
B. rectus femoris muscle
C. tensor muscle
D. iliopsoas muscle
E. urethra
F. greater trochanter
G. vagina
H. levator ani muscle
I. rectum
J. gluteal maximus muscle
K. obturator internus muscle
L. obturator foramen
M. head of femur
N. obturator externus muscle
O. pectineus muscle
P. superior ramus of pubic bone
Q. body of pubic bone
R. symphysis pubis

Exercise 7-21: Labeling

A. sartorius muscle
B. rectus femoris muscle
C. tensor muscle
D. iliopsoas muscle
E. symphysis pubis
F. gluteal maximus muscle
G. ischial tuberosity
H. levator ani muscle
I. rectum
J. vagina
K. urethra

Exercise 7-22: Labeling

A. sartorius muscle
B. rectus femoris muscle
C. iliopsoas muscle

D. urethra
E. vagina
F. gluteal maximus muscle
G. ischial tuberosity
H. inferior ramus of pubic bone

Exercise 7-23: Labeling

A. rectus abdominis muscle
B. iliacus muscle
C. gluteal medius muscle
D. SI joint
E. gluteal maximus muscle
F. ilium
G. sacral promontory
H. psoas muscle
I. lateral muscles

Exercise 7-24: Labeling

A. rectus abdominis muscle
B. ovary
C. psoas muscle
D. iliacus muscle
E. SI joint
F. sacrum
G. gluteal maximus muscle
H. ilium
I. gluteal medius muscle
J. lateral muscles

Exercise 7-25: Labeling

A. rectus abdominis muscle
B. ovary
C. iliopsoas muscle
D. ilium
E. SI joint
F. sacrum
G. gluteal maximus muscle
H. gluteal medius muscle
I. gluteal minimus muscle
J. ovary

Exercise 7-26: Labeling

A. rectus abdominis muscle
B. iliopsoas muscle
C. gluteal maximus muscle
D. gluteal medius muscle
E. gluteal minimus muscle
F. external iliac vein
G. external iliac artery
H. ovary
I. lateral muscles

Exercise 7-27: Labeling

A. rectus abdominis muscle
B. external iliac artery
C. external iliac vein
D. hip bone
E. piriformis muscle
F. gluteal maximus muscle
G. sigmoid colon
H. gluteal medius muscle
I. gluteal minimus muscle
J. iliopsoas muscle
K. lateral muscles

Exercise 7-28: Labeling

A. iliopsoas muscle
B. rectum
C. gluteal maximus muscle
D. piriformis muscle
E. external iliac vein
F. external iliac artery
G. rectus abdominis muscle

Exercise 7-29: Labeling

A. iliopsoas muscle
B. rectum
C. gluteal maximus muscle
D. piriformis muscle
E. external iliac vein
F. external iliac artery
G. rectus abdominus muscle

Exercise 7-30: Labeling

A. iliopsoas muscle
B. external iliac vein
C. cervix of uterus
D. rectum
E. gluteal maximus muscle
F. acetabulum
G. bladder
H. external iliac artery
I. rectus abdominis muscle

Exercise 7-31: Labeling

A. external iliac vein
B. bladder
C. head of femur
D. acetabulum
E. levator ani muscle
F. gluteal maximus muscle
G. rectum

H. cervix of uterus
I. iliopsoas muscle
J. external iliac artery
K. rectus abdominis muscle

Exercise 7-32: Labeling

A. external iliac artery
B. bladder
C. pubic bone
D. vagina
E. ischium
F. levator ani muscle
G. gluteal maximus muscle
H. rectum
I. head of femur
J. acetabulum
K. external iliac vein
L. rectus abdominis muscle

Exercise 7-33: Labeling

A. bladder
B. femur
C. vagina
D. rectum
E. levator ani muscle
F. gluteal maximus muscle
G. ischium
H. obturator internus muscle
I. pubic bone

Exercise 7-34: Labeling

A. symphysis pubis
B. urethra
C. vagina
D. rectum
E. levator ani muscle
F. gluteal maximus muscle
G. ischial tuberosity
H. obturator internus muscle
I. obturator externus muscle

Exercise 7-35: Labeling

A. symphysis pubis
B. urethra
C. vagina
D. anus
E. levator ani muscle
F. gluteal maximus muscle
G. ischial tuberosity
H. body of pubic bone

Exercise 7-36: Labeling

A. rectus femoris muscle
B. urethra
C. vagina
D. gluteal maximus muscle
E. anus
F. inferior ramus of pubic bone
G. iliopsoas muscle
H. sartorius muscle

Exercise 7-37: Labeling

A. gluteal maximus muscle

Exercise 7-38: Labeling

A. gluteal maximus muscle
B. body of ilium
C. acetabulum
D. body of ischium
E. ischial tuberosity
F. obturator externus muscle
G. head of femur
H. pubic bone
I. iliopsoas muscle
J. iliacus muscle

Exercise 7-39: Labeling

A. gluteal medius muscle
B. ilium
C. piriformis muscle
D. gluteal maximus muscle
E. ischium
F. ischial tuberosity
G. obturator externus muscle
H. pubic bone
I. pectineus muscle
J. femur
K. iliopsoas muscle
L. iliacus muscle
M. psoas muscle
N. rectus abdominis muscle

Exercise 7-40: Labeling

A. ilium
B. piriformis muscle
C. obturator internus muscle
D. gluteal maximus muscle
E. ischial ramus
F. obturator externus muscle
G. pectineus muscle
H. pubic bone
I. rectus abdominis muscle

J. iliacus muscle
K. psoas muscle

Exercise 7-41: Labeling

A. ilium
B. sacroiliac joint
C. sacrum
D. piriformis muscle
E. gluteal maximus muscle
F. obturator internus muscle
G. obturator externus muscle
H. rectus abdominis muscle
I. psoas muscle

Exercise 7-42: Labeling

A. sacrum
B. gluteal maximus muscle
C. bladder
D. rectus abdominis muscle
E. psoas muscle

Exercise 7-43: Labeling

A. sacrum
B. gluteal maximus muscle
C. pubis
D. bladder
E. rectus abdominis muscle
F. small intestine

Exercise 7-44: Labeling

A. sacral segment
B. pubis
C. bladder
D. rectus abdominis muscle
E. aorta
F. IVC

Exercise 7-45: Labeling

A. sacrum
B. vagina
C. anus
D. urethra
E. pubis
F. bladder
G. rectus abdominis muscle

Exercise 7-46: Labeling

A. sacrum
B. rectum
C. cervix

D. vagina
E. anus
F. urethra
G. symphysis pubis
H. bladder
I. uterine cavity
J. rectus abdominis muscle

Exercise 7-47: Labeling

A. sacrum
B. rectum
C. cervix
D. vagina
E. pubis
F. bladder
G. rectus abdominis muscle
H. uterine cavity

Exercise 7-48: Labeling

A. sacral segment
B. pubis
C. bladder
D. rectus abdominis muscle

Exercise 7-49: Labeling

A. sacrum
B. gluteal maximus muscle
C. pubis
D. bladder
E. rectus abdominis muscle

Exercise 7-50: Labeling

A. sacrum
B. gluteal maximus muscle
C. rectus abdominis muscle
D. psoas muscle

Exercise 7-51: Labeling

A. ilium
B. sacroiliac (SI) joint
C. sacrum
D. gluteal maximus muscle
E. rectus abdominis muscle
F. psoas muscle

Exercise 7-52: Labeling

A. ilium
B. piriformis muscle
C. gluteal maximus muscle
D. obturator internus muscle

E. ischial ramus
F. obturator externus muscle
G. pectineus muscle
H. pubic bone
I. rectus abdominis muscle
J. psoas muscle

Exercise 7-53: Labeling

A. ilium
B. gluteal maximus muscle
C. body of ischium
D. ischial tuberosity
E. obturator externus muscle
F. pectineus muscle
G. pubic bone
H. iliopsoas muscle
I. iliacus muscle
J. psoas muscle

Exercise 7-54: Labeling

A. gluteal medius muscle
B. gluteal minimus muscle
C. gluteal maximus muscle
D. body of ilium
E. acetabulum
F. body of ischium
G. ischial tuberosity
H. obturator externus muscle
I. head of femur
J. pubic bone
K. iliopsoas muscle
L. iliacus muscle

CHAPTER 8: VERTEBRAL COLUMN

Exercise 8-1: Labeling

A. superior articular process
B. transverse process
C. inferior articular process
D. inferior vertebral notch
E. superior vertebral notch
F. spinous process
G. apophyseal joint
H. intervertebral foramen
I. annulus fibrosus
J. nucleus pulposus
K. intervertebral disc

Exercise 8-2: Matching

1. b
2. d
3. e
4. a
5. c

Exercise 8-3: Identification

1. transverse process
2. transverse process
3. spinous process
4. superior articulating process
5. superior articulating process
6. inferior articulating process
7. inferior articulating process

Exercise 8-4: Completion

(Terms listed in the order they appear.)
foramen magnum
medulla oblongata
cervical
lumbar
vertebral canal
conus medullaris
cauda equina
coccyx
filium terminale
pia mater
spinal nerves
cervical
coccygeal

Exercise 8-5: Matching

1. b
2. a
3. c
4. e
5. d

Exercise 8-6: Labeling

A. cervical spinal nerves
B. thoracic spinal nerves
C. lumbar spinal nerves
D. sacral spinal nerves
E. filium terminale
F. coccygeal nerve
G. cauda equina
H. conus medullaris
I. lumbar enlargement

J. dura mater
K. cervical enlargement

Exercise 8-7: Labeling

A. spinal cord/medulla oblongata
B. foramen magnum
C. occipital bone
D. superior articulating facet C1

Exercise 8-8: Labeling

A. atlas C1
B. transverse process
C. vertebral artery
D. transverse foramen
E. lateral mass
F. posterior arch C1
G. spinal cord
H. odontoid process C2
I. anterior arch C1

Exercise 8-9: Labeling

A. transverse foramen
B. vertebral artery
C. spinal cord
D. spinous process
E. ligamentum nuchae
F. lamina
G. vertebral arch
H. vertebral foramen
I. pedicle
J. body C2

Exercise 8-10: Labeling

A. vertebral artery
B. transverse foramen
C. spinal cord
D. spinous process
E. lamina
F. vertebral foramen
G. pedicle
H. body

Exercise 8-11: Labeling

A. spinal cord
B. lamina
C. pedicle
D. body

Exercise 8-12: Labeling

A. intervertebral foramen
B. spinal cord

C. ligamentum nuchae
D. bifid spinous process
E. lamina
F. body

Exercise 8-13: Labeling

A. intervertebral disk
B. intervertebral foramen
C. ligamentum flava
D. superior articulating process L5
E. inferior articulating process L4
F. supraspinous ligament
G. spinous process
H. zygoapophyseal joint
I. posterior longitudinal ligament
J. nucleus pulposus
K. annulus fibrosus
L. anterior longitudinal ligament

Exercise 8-14: Labeling

A. anterior longitudinal ligament
B. posterior longitudinal ligament
C. transverse process
D. vertebral foramen
E. inferior articulating process L4
F. spinous process L4
G. supraspinous ligament
H. ligamentum flava
I. superior articulating process L5
J. zygoapophyseal joint
K. pedicle
L. body L5

Exercise 8-15: Labeling

A. anterior longitudinal ligament
B. transverse process
C. neural arch
D. cauda equina
E. lamina
F. supraspinous ligament
G. spinous process L5
H. vertebral foramen
I. pedicle
J. body L5

Exercise 8-16: Labeling

A. body L5
B. superior articulating process S1
C. inferior articulating process L5
D. supraspinous ligament

E. spinous process
F. intervertebral foramen

Exercise 8-17: Labeling

A. intervertebral foramen
B. spinous process
C. inferior articulating process L5
D. superior articulating process S1
E. body L5

Exercise 8-18: Labeling

A. sacrum

Exercise 8-19: Labeling

A. spinal cord
B. central canal—CSF
C. posterior longitudinal ligament
D. ligamentum flava
E. conus medullaris
F. supraspinous ligament
G. cauda equina
H. anterior longitudinal ligament
I. annulus fibrosus
J. intervertebral disk
K. body
L. nucleus pulposus

Exercise 8-20: Labeling

A. pedicle
B. superior articulating process
C. inferior articulating process
D. zygoapophyseal joint
E. intervertebral foramen
F. annulus fibrosus
G. body
H. nucleus pulposus
I. intervertebral disk

Exercise 8-21: Labeling

A. anterior longitudinal ligament
B. posterior longitudinal ligament
C. transverse process
D. ligamentum flava
E. cauda equina
F. pedicle
G. vertebral foramen
H. body L3

Exercise 8-22: Labeling

A. anterior longitudinal ligament
B. posterior longitudinal ligament

C. ligamentum flava
D. spinous process L3
E. supraspinous ligament
F. lamina
G. cauda equina
H. intervertebral foramen
I. body L3

Exercise 8-23: Labeling

A. intervertebral disk between L3/4
B. nucleus pulposus
C. PLL
D. cauda equina
E. supraspinous ligament
F. spinous process
G. ligamentum flava
H. intervertebral foramen
I. annulus fibrosus
J. ALL

Exercise 8-24: Labeling

A. ALL
B. annulus fibrosus
C. cauda equina
D. ligamentum flava
E. spinous process L3
F. supraspinous ligament
G. inferior articulating process L3
H. superior articulating process L4
I. zygoapophyseal joint
J. PLL
K. nucleus pulposus
L. intervertebral disk

Exercise 8-25: Labeling

A. ALL
B. cauda equina
C. zygoapophyseal joint
D. spinous process
E. supraspinous ligament
F. inferior articulating process L3
G. superior articulating process L4
H. ligamentum flava
I. PLL
J. body L4

Exercise 8-26: Labeling

A. ALL
B. pedicle
C. transverse process

D. ligamentum flava
E. superior articulating process L4
F. cauda equina
G. PLL
H. body L4

CHAPTER 9: UPPER EXTREMITY

Exercise 9-1: Matching

1. b
2. d
3. a
4. a

Exercise 9-2: Term Identification

1. D
2. C
3. B
4. A

Exercise 9-3: Identification

1. skull
2. auditory ossicles
3. hyoid bone
4. sternum
5. ribs
6. vertebral column

Exercise 9-4: Identification

1. shoulder girdle
2. pelvic girdle
3. upper extremity
4. lower extremity

Exercise 9-5: Matching

1. a
2. d
3. e
4. b
5. c

Exercise 9-6: Identification

1. A
2. A
3. A
4. A
5. B

6. A
7. B
8. B
9. A
10. B
11. A
12. B
13. A

Exercise 9-7: Identification

1. B
2. B
3. B
4. A
5. A
6. C
7. C
8. B
9. A
10. A

Exercise 9-8: Identification

1. subscapularis
2. supraspinatus
3. infraspinatus
4. teres minor

Exercise 9-9: Identification

1. B
2. B
3. B

Exercise 9-10: Identification

1. A
2. B
3. C
4. C
5. B
6. C
7. B

Exercise 9-11: Sorting

a

Exercise 9-12: Matching

1. c
2. d
3. b
4. a

Exercise 9-13: Labeling

A. acromioclavicular ligaments
B. clavicle
C. coracoacromial ligament
D. coracohumeral ligament
E. coracoid process
F. subcoracoid bursa
G. subscapularis bursa
H. glenohumeral ligament
I. transverse humeral ligament
J. subscaularis tendon (cut)
K. greater and lesser tubercules of humerus
L. subacromial/subdeltoid bursa
M. acromion

Exercise 9-14: Labeling

A. humerus
B. medial epicondyle
C. ulnar collateral ligament
D. ulna
E. radius
F. annular ligament of radius
G. radial collateral ligament
H. lateral epicondyle
I. joint capsule

Exercise 9-15: Labeling

A. radius
B. dorsal radiocarpal ligament
C. lunate bone
D. scaphoid bone
E. capitate bone
F. radial collateral ligament
G. trapezoid bone
H. trapezium bone
I. metacarpal bones
J. hamate bone
K. triquetrum bone
L. dorsal ulnocarpal ligament
M. ulna collateral ligament
N. ulna

Exercise 9-16: Term Identification

1. supinator longus muscle
2. synovial joint
3. posterior ligament
4. bicipital groove
5. anterior ligament

6. external ligament
7. glenohumeral joint
8. internal ligament

Exercise 9-17: Labeling

A. acromioclavicular (AC) joint
B. acromion of scapula
C. spine of scapula
D. acromial end of clavicle

Exercise 9-18: Labeling

A. bicipital groove of humerus
B. head of humerus
C. greater tubercle of humerus
D. scapula
E. neck of scapula
F. glenoid fossa of scapula
G. coracoid process of scapula
H. lesser tubercle of humerus

Exercise 9-19: Labeling

A. shaft of humerus
B. axillary border of scapula
C. ribs

Exercise 9-20: Labeling

A. pectoralis muscle
B. coracoid process of scapula
C. anterior labrum
D. subscapularis muscle
E. infraspinatus muscle
F. deltoid muscle
G. posterior labrum
H. glenoid fossa of scapula
I. head of humerus
J. coracohumeral ligament

Exercise 9-21: Labeling

A. subacromial/subdeltoid bursa
B. supraspinatus muscle
C. superior labrum
D. scapula
E. glenoid fossa of scapula
F. inferior labrum
G. anatomical neck of humerus
H. greater tubercle of humerus
I. head of humerus
J. deltoid muscle
K. rotator cuff
L. acromion of scapula

Exercise 9-22: Labeling

A. infraspinatus muscle
B. deltoid muscle
C. head of humerus
D. supraspinatus muscle
E. acromion

Exercise 9-23: Labeling

A. pronator teres muscle
B. medial humerus
C. distal humerus
D. triceps muscle
E. brachioradialis muscle
F. lateral humerus
G. brachialis muscle
H. biceps brachii muscle

Exercise 9-24: Labeling

A. pronator teres muscle
B. medial epicondyle of humerus
C. olecranon process of ulna
D. lateral epicondyle of humerus
E. brachioradialis muscle
F. olecranon fossa of humerus
G. brachialis muscle

Exercise 9-25: Labeling

A. pronator teres muscle
B. medial epicondyle of humerus
C. olecranon process of ulna
D. olecranon fossa of humerus
E. lateral epicondyle of humerus
F. extensor carpi radialis longus muscle
G. brachioradialis muscle
H. brachialis muscle

Exercise 9-26: Labeling

A. pronator teres muscle
B. medial condyle of humerus
C. olecranon process of ulna
D. anconeus muscle
E. extensor carpi radialis muscle
F. lateral condyle of humerus
G. brachioradialis muscle
H. brachialis muscle

Exercise 9-27: Labeling

A. pronator teres muscle
B. flexor muscle

C. brachialis muscle
D. ulna
E. anconeus muscle
F. annular ligament
G. radial head
H. extensor carpi radialis muscle
I. brachioradialis muscle
J. supinator muscle

Exercise 9-28: Labeling

A. brachialis muscle
B. brachioradialis muscle
C. extensor carpi radialis muscle
D. lateral epicondyle of humerus
E. olecranon process of ulna
F. olecranon fossa of humerus
G. medial epicondyle of humerus
H. pronator teres muscle

Exercise 9-29: Labeling

A. triceps brachii muscle
B. medial epicondyle of humerus
C. medial collateral ligament
D. trochlea of humerus
E. coronoid process of ulna
F. radial notch of ulna
G. flexor muscles
H. lateral collateral ligament
I. extensor muscle
J. radial tuberosity
K. brachioradialis muscle
L. neck of radius
M. head of radius
N. capitulum of humerus
O. lateral epicondyle of humerus
P. coronoid fossa of humerus
Q. triceps brachii muscle
R. shaft of humerus

Exercise 9-30: Labeling

A. triceps brachii muscle
B. medial epicondyle of humerus
C. olecranon process of ulna
D. ulna
E. flexor muscles
F. supinator muscle
G. head of radius
H. lateral epicondyle of humerus
I. olecranon fossa of humerus
J. triceps brachii muscle
K. shaft of humerus

Exercise 9-31: Labeling

A. distal radius
B. distal ulna

Exercise 9-32: Labeling

A. scaphoid
B. lunate
C. pisiform

Exercise 9-33: Labeling

A. first metacarpal
B. trapezium
C. capitate
D. hamate
E. triquetrum
F. trapezoid

Exercise 9-34: Labeling

A. flexor muscle tendons
B. distal radius
C. extensor muscle tendons
D. distal ulna

Exercise 9-35: Labeling

A. flexor retinaculum manus
B. flexor muscle tendons
C. trapezium
D. trapezoid
E. extensor muscle tendons
F. capitate
G. hamate
H. carpal tunnel

Exercise 9-36: Labeling

A. scaphoid
B. trapezium
C. flexor muscle tendons
D. pisiform

Exercise 9-37: Labeling

A. distal radius
B. styloid process of radius
C. lunate
D. scaphoid
E. trapezium
F. trapezoid
G. hamate
H. capitate
I. pisiform
J. triquetrum

K. styloid process of ulna
L. distal ulna

Exercise 9-38: Labeling

A. distal radius
B. extensor muscle tendons
C. scaphoid
D. proximal metacarpal
E. capitate
F. flexor muscle tendons

Exercise 9-39: Labeling

A. triquetrum
B. extensor muscle tendons
C. proximal metacarpal
D. hamate
E. flexor muscle tendons
F. pisiform

CHAPTER 10: LOWER EXTREMITY

Exercise 10-1: Identification

A. femur
B. patella
C. fibula
D. tibia
E. tarsal bones
F. metatarsals
G. phalanges

Exercise 10-2: Identification

1. A
2. A
3. B
4. C
5. A
6. B
7. A
8. C

Exercise 10-3: Identification

A. talus or astragalus
B. calcaneus or os calcis
C. cuboid
D. navicular
E. first or medial cuneiform
F. second or intermediate cuneiform
G. third or lateral cuneiform

Exercise 10-4: Term Identification

1. mortise joint
2. hallux
3. os calcis
4. thigh
5. medial cuneiform
6. astragalus

Exercise 10-5: Identification

1. gastrocnemius
2. soleus

Exercise 10-6: Matching

1. b
2. b
3. b

Exercise 10-7: Matching

1. d
2. a
3. d

Exercise 10-8: Identification

1. C
2. C
3. C
4. B
5. A
6. A
7. C
8. B
9. A

Exercise 10-9: Identification

1. C
2. D
3. B
4. B
5. B
6. C
7. A
8. A
9. D

Exercise 10-10: Identification

1. D
2. C

3. A
4. B

Exercise 10-11: Completion

quadriceps femoris muscle

Exercise 10-12: Identification

A. biceps femoris
B. semimembranosus
C. semitendinosus

Exercise 10-13: Identification

1. A
2. A
3. B
4. A

Exercise 10-14: Identification

1. A
2. B
3. C
4. B
5. B

Exercise 10-15: Identification

1. Achilles
2. sartorius
3. femur or thigh

Exercise 10-16: Labeling

A. superior pubic ramus
B. iliopectineal bursa
C. pubofemoral ligament
D. lesser trochanter
E. intertrochanteric line
F. iliofemoral ligament
G. greater trochanter
H. anterior inferior iliac spine
I. anterior superior iliac spine

Exercise 10-17: Labeling

A. lateral condyle of femur
B. anterior cruciate ligament
C. fibular collateral ligament
D. lateral meniscus
E. tibial tuberosity
F. fibula

G. tibia
H. transverse ligament
I. medial meniscus
J. tibial collateral ligament
K. medial condyle of femur
L. posterior cruciate ligament
M. femur

Exercise 10-18: Labeling

A. tibia
B. medial malleolus of tibia
C. posterior process of talus
D. posterior talocalcaneal ligament
E. Achilles tendon (cut)
F. medial talocalcaneal ligament
G. sustentaculum tali
H. plantar (spring) ligament
I. first metatarsal bone
J. first cuneiform bone
K. navicular bone
L. dorsal talonavicular ligament
M. medial (deltoid) ligament

Exercise 10-19: Labeling

A. tensor muscle
B. ilium
C. gluteal minimus muscle
D. gluteal medius muscle
E. gluteal maximus muscle
F. sacrum
G. piriformis muscle
H. iliopsoas muscle
I. sartorius muscle

Exercise 10-20: Labeling

A. tensor muscle
B. gluteal minimus muscle
C. gluteal medius muscle
D. gluteal maximus muscle
E. piriformis muscle
F. obturator internus muscle
G. roof of the acetabulum
H. iliopsoas muscle
I. sartorius muscle

Exercise 10-21: Labeling

A. sartorius muscle
B. tensor muscle
C. head of femur

D. gluteal maximus muscle
E. sacrum
F. acetabulum
G. iliopsoas muscle

Exercise 10-22: Labeling

A. sartorius muscle
B. tensor muscle
C. rectus femoris muscle
D. greater trochanter of the femur
E. gluteal maximus muscle
F. ischial spine
G. superior gemellus muscle
H. head of the femur
I. acetabulum
J. fovea capitis
K. iliopsoas muscle

Exercise 10-23: Labeling

A. sartorius muscle
B. iliopsoas muscle
C. tensor muscle
D. rectus femoris muscle
E. head of femur
F. greater trochanter
G. superior gemellus muscle
H. gluteal maximus muscle
I. ischial spine
J. obturator internus muscle
K. ischium
L. superior ramus of pubic bone
M. body of pubic bone
N. symphysis pubis
O. pectineus muscle

Exercise 10-24: Labeling

A. sartorius muscle
B. tensor muscle
C. rectus femoris muscle
D. iliopsoas muscle
E. vastus lateralis muscle
F. neck of femur
G. quadratus femoris muscle
H. greater trochanter of femur
I. gluteal maximus muscle
J. ischium
K. obturator internus muscle
L. obturator externus muscle
M. body of pubic bone
N. pectineus muscle

Exercise 10-25: Labeling

A. sartorius muscle
B. rectus femoris muscle
C. tensor muscle
D. iliopsoas muscle
E. vastus lateralis muscle
F. neck of femur
G. obturator externus muscle
H. quadratus femoris muscle
I. gluteal maximus muscle
J. ischial tuberosity
K. obturator internus muscle
L. inferior ramus of pubic bone
M. symphysis pubis

Exercise 10-26: Labeling

A. rectus femoris muscle
B. tensor muscle
C. vastus lateralis muscle
D. femoral shaft
E. quadratus femoris muscle
F. biceps femoris tendon
G. gluteal maximus muscle
H. ischial tuberosity
I. adductor magnus muscle
J. adductor brevis muscle
K. adductor longus muscle
L. sartorius muscle

Exercise 10-27: Labeling

A. tensor muscle
B. acetabular roof
C. obturator internus muscle
D. piriformis muscle
E. gluteal maximus muscle
F. gluteal medius muscle
G. gluteal minimus muscle
H. iliopsoas muscle
I. sartorius muscle

Exercise 10-28: Labeling

A. iliopsoas muscle
B. tensor muscle
C. acetabulum
D. ligament of head of femur
E. greater trochanter
F. ischium
G. superior gemellus muscle
H. gluteal maximus muscle
I. gluteal medius muscle

J. obturator internus muscle
K. acetabular fossa
L. fovea capitis
M. head of femur
N. sartorius muscle

Exercise 10-29: Labeling

A. rectus femoris muscle
B. tensor muscle
C. iliopsoas muscle
D. gluteal minimus muscle
E. neck of femur
F. greater trochanter
G. obturator internus muscle
H. superior gemellus muscle
I. gluteal maximus muscle
J. gluteal medius muscle
K. ischium
L. acetabulum
M. head of femur
N. acetabular fossa
O. sartorius muscle

Exercise 10-30: Labeling

A. rectus femoris muscle
B. tensor muscle
C. iliopsoas muscle
D. head of femur
E. ischium
F. superior gemellus muscle
G. obturator internus muscle
H. gluteal maximus muscle
I. ischial spine
J. gluteal medius muscle
K. greater trochanter
L. acetabulum
M. gluteal minimus muscle
N. sartorius muscle

Exercise 10-31: Labeling

A. gluteal maximus muscle
B. gluteal medius muscle
C. acetabulum
D. head of femur
E. symphysis pubis
F. vastus lateralis muscle
G. body of pubic bone
H. superior ramus of pubic bone
I. iliopsoas muscle
J. iliacus muscle
K. ilium
L. psoas muscle

Exercise 10-32: Labeling

A. gluteal maximus muscle
B. gluteal medius muscle
C. acetabulum
D. labrum
E. head of femur
F. fovea capitis
G. greater trochanter
H. neck of femur
I. transverse ligament
J. vastus lateralis muscle
K. gracilis muscle
L. adductor muscle
M. obturator externus muscle
N. obturator internus muscle
O. ligamentum teres femoris
P. acetabular fossa
Q. iliofemoral ligament
R. iliopsoas muscle
S. iliacus muscle
T. ilium
U. psoas muscle

Exercise 10-33: Labeling

A. acetabulum
B. head of femur
C. greater trochanter
D. neck of femur
E. gemellus muscle
F. quadratus femoris muscle
G. vastus lateralis muscle
H. adductor muscle
I. ischium
J. obturator internus
K. body of ilium

Exercise 10-34: Labeling

A. gluteal maximus muscle
B. intertrochanteric crest
C. lesser trochanter
D. quadratus femoris muscle
E. adductor muscle
F. vastus intermedius muscle
G. rectus femoris muscle
H. greater trochanter

Exercise 10-35: Labeling

A. gluteal minimus muscle
B. gluteal medius muscle
C. gluteal maximus muscle

D. acetabulum
E. transverse ligament
F. sartorius muscle
G. iliofemoral ligament
H. femoral head
I. iliopsoas muscle
J. labrum
K. ilium

Exercise 10-36: Labeling

A. vastus lateralis muscle
B. distal femur
C. biceps femoris muscle
D. semimembranosus muscle
E. sartorius muscle
F. vastus medialis muscle
G. suprapatellar bursa

Exercise 10-37: Labeling

A. articular cartilage of patella
B. lateral patellar retinaculum
C. femur
D. biceps femoris muscle
E. semimembranosus muscle
F. sartorius muscle
G. vastus medialis muscle
H. medial patellar retinaculum
I. base of patella

Exercise 10-38: Labeling

A. articular capsule
B. anterior cruciate ligament
C. lateral condyle of femur
D. biceps femoris muscle
E. plantaris muscle
F. lateral head of gastrocnemius
   muscle
G. medial head of gastrocnemius
   muscle
H. semimembranosus muscle
I. sartorius muscle
J. posterior cruciate ligament
K. medial condyle of femur
L. intercondylar fossa
M. articular cartilage of femur
N. patella

Exercise 10-39: Labeling

A. lateral collateral ligament
B. lateral condyle of femur

C. anterior cruciate ligament
D. plantaris muscle
E. lateral head of gastrocnemius
   muscle
F. medial head of gastrocnemius
   muscle
G. sartorius muscle
H. posterior cruciate ligament
I. medial condyle of femur
J. intercondylar fossa
K. medial collateral ligament
L. apex of patella

Exercise 10-40: Labeling

A. patellar ligament
B. lateral collateral ligament
C. lateral condyle of femur
D. plantaris muscle
E. lateral head of gastrocnemius
   muscle
F. medial head of gastrocnemius
   muscle
G. medial condyle of femur
H. intercondylar tubercle
I. medial collateral ligament
J. infrapatellar fat pad

Exercise 10-41: Labeling

A. patellar ligament
B. lateral condyle of tibia
C. popliteus muscle
D. plantaris muscle
E. lateral head of gastrocnemius
   muscle
F. medial head of gastrocnemius
   muscle
G. medial condyle of tibia
H. tibia
I. infrapatellar fat pad

Exercise 10-42: Labeling

A. patellar ligament
B. proximal fibula
C. plantaris muscle
D. lateral head of gastrocnemius
   muscle
E. medial head of gastrocnemius
   muscle
F. semitendinosus muscle tendon
G. popliteus muscle

H. semimembranosus muscle tendon
I. gracilis muscle tendon
J. proximal tibia

Exercise 10-43: Labeling

A. patella
B. intercondylar fossa
C. lateral condyle of femur
D. anterior cruciate ligament
E. popliteal artery
F. biceps femoris muscle
G. popliteal vein
H. lateral head of gastrocnemius muscle
I. semimembranosus muscle
J. medial head of gastrocnemius muscle
K. sartorius muscle
L. posterior cruciate ligament
M. medial condyle of femur
N. articular cartilage

Exercise 10-44: Labeling

A. vastus medialis muscle
B. medial collateral ligament
C. medial meniscus
D. intercondylar eminence
E. tibia
F. tibial plateau
G. lateral meniscus
H. articular cartilage of femur
I. femur
J. vastus lateralis muscle

Exercise 10-45: Labeling

A. vastus medialis muscle
B. posterior cruciate ligament
C. medial collateral ligament
D. medial condyle of femur
E. medial meniscus
F. medial condyle of tibia
G. tibia
H. lateral condyle of tibia
I. lateral collateral ligament
J. lateral meniscus
K. anterior cruciate ligament
L. lateral condyle of femur
M. intercondylar fossa
N. femur
O. vastus lateralis muscle

Exercise 10-46: Labeling

A. semimembranosus muscle
B. semitendinosus muscle
C. distal femur
D. gastrocnemius muscle
E. posterior cruciate ligament
F. popliteus muscle
G. proximal tibia
H. anterior cruciate ligament
I. infrapatellar fat pad
J. apex of patella
K. patellar ligament
L. articulating cartilage
M. prepatellar bursa
N. base of patella
O. suprapatellar bursa
P. quadriceps muscle tendon

Exercise 10-47: Labeling

A. semimembranosus muscle
B. joint capsule
C. gastrocnemius muscle
D. medial meniscus
E. patellar ligament
F. medial condyle of tibia
G. articular cartilage
H. infrapatellar fat pad
I. medial condyle of femur
J. vastus medialis muscle

Exercise 10-48: Labeling

A. fibula
B. tibia

Exercise 10-49: Labeling

A. extensor hallucis longus muscle tendon
B. extensor digitorum longus muscle tendon
C. peroneus tertius muscle
D. lateral malleolus of fibula
E. flexor hallucis longus muscle tendon
F. flexor digitorum longus muscle tendon
G. tibialis posterior muscle tendon
H. trochlea of talus
I. medial malleolus of tibia
J. tibialis anterior muscle tendon

Exercise 10-50: Labeling

A. extensor digitorum longus muscle tendon
B. peroneus tertius muscle
C. lateral malleolus of fibula
D. peroneus longus muscle tendon
E. peroneus brevis muscle tendon
F. calcaneus
G. flexor hallucis longus muscle tendon
H. posterior process of talus
I. flexor digitorum longus muscle tendon
J. tibialis posterior muscle tendon
K. medial malleolus of tibia
L. tibialis anterior muscle tendon
M. extensor hallucis longus muscle tendon

Exercise 10-51: Labeling

A. lateral malleolus of fibula
B. calcaneus
C. posterior process of talus

Exercise 10-52: Labeling

A. lateral malleolus of fibula
B. posterior process of talus
C. calcaneus
D. sustentaculum tali

Exercise 10-53: Labeling

A. lateral malleolus of fibula
B. calcaneus
C. sustentaculum tali of calcaneus
D. spring ligament
E. deltoid ligament
F. head of talus
G. navicular

Exercise 10-54: Labeling

A. lateral process of talus
B. calcaneus
C. sustentaculum tali
D. navicular
E. head of talus

Exercise 10-55: Labeling

A. talus
B. calcaneus
C. navicular

Exercise 10-56: Labeling

A. calcaneus
B. navicular
C. first (medial) cuneiform

Exercise 10-57: Labeling

A. third (lateral) cuneiform
B. cuboid
C. calcaneus
D. first (medial) cuneiform
E. second (intermediate)
   cuneiform

Exercise 10-58: Labeling

A. tibialis anterior
B. medial malleolus of tibia
C. tibiotalar ligament
D. tibialis posterior
E. flexor hallucis longus
F. Achilles tendon
G. peroneus brevis

H. peroneus longus
I. posterior talofibular ligament
J. lateral malleolus of fibula
K. talus
L. anterior talofibular ligament
M. extensor digitorum longus
N. extensor hallucis longus

Exercise 10-59: Labeling

A. articular cartilage
B. mortise joint
C. lateral malleolus of fibula
D. calcaneus
E. sustentaculum tali
F. deltoid ligament
G. trochlea of talus
H. medial malleolus of tibia
I. tibia

Exercise 10-60: Labeling

A. tibia
B. posterior tibiofibular ligament

C. Achilles tendon
D. sinus tarsi
E. calcaneus
F. cuboid
G. interosseous talocalcaneal
   ligament
H. trochlea of talus
I. tibiotalar joint
J. extensor hallucis longus muscle

Exercise 10-61: Labeling

A. tibialis posterior muscle
B. tibiotalar joint
C. interosseous talocalcaneal
   ligament
D. calcaneus
E. subtalar joint
F. intermediate cuneiform
G. navicular
H. head of talus
I. trochlea of talus
J. tibia

Appendix B
Word Lists

Chapter 2: Head

Blood Vessels

Circle of Willis
  Communicating arteries, ant., post.
Common carotid arteries, R/L
  External carotid arteries
  Internal carotid arteries
    Ant. cerebral arteries
    Middle cerebral arteries
Vertebral arteries
  Basilar artery
    Post. cerebral arteries

Brain

Forebrain
  Cerebrum
    Basal ganglia
      Amygdaloid nucleus
      Claustrum
      Corpus striatum
        Caudate nucleus
          Head, body, tail
        Lentiform nucleus
          Globus pallidus
          Putamen
    Internal capsule
    Centrum semiovale—white matter
    Corpus callosum
      Body or trunk
      Genu
      Splenium
    Cortex—gray matter
      Gyrus or convolution
      Sulcus

Fissures
  Central
  Longitudinal
  Sylvian or lat.
  Transverse
  Falx cerebelli
  Falx cerebri
  Tentorium cerebelli
Hemispheres, R/L
Lobes
  Central lobe or insula
  Frontal
  Occipital
  Parietal
  Temporal
Diencephalon
  Hypothalamus
    Infundibulum
  Thalamus
    Intermediate mass

Midbrain

Peduncles
Quadrigeminal plate/tectum/
  Corpora quadrigemina
    Colliculi, R/L sup. and inf.

Hindbrain

Cerebellum
  Ant. cerebellar notch
  Hemispheres, R/L
  Post. cerebellar notch
  Vermis
Medulla oblongata
Pons

Cisterns
- Cistern pontine
- Cisterna magna
- Quadrigeminal cistern

Cranium
- Cranial bones
  - Ethmoid
    - Cribriform plate
    - Crista galli
  - Frontal
    - Ethmoidal notch
    - Horizontal/orbital section
    - Squamous portion
  - Occipital
    - Foramen magnum
  - Parietal
  - Sphenoid
    - Ant. clinoids
    - Dorsum sellae
    - Post. clinoids
    - Pterygoid processes
    - Sella turcica
  - Temporal bone
    - Mastoid portion
    - Petrous portion/pyramids/ridge
    - Temporomandibular fossa
- Diploe

Dural Sinuses
- Ant. sup. sagittal sinus
- Post. sup. sagittal sinus

Miscellaneous
- Optic chiasma
- Optic nerve
- Pineal gland
- Pituitary gland
- Scalp
- Spinal cord
- White matter

Ventricles
- Lateral
  - Body
  - Fornix
  - Frontal/ant. horn
  - Interventricular foramen/foramen of Monro
  - Occipital/post. horn
  - Septum pellucidum
  - Temporal/inf. horn
    - Collateral trigone/choroid plexus
- Third ventricle
  - Cerebral aqueduct/Sylvian aqueduct/Aqueduct of Sylvius
- Fourth ventricle
  - Foramen of Magendie/median aperture
  - Foramina of Luschka/lat. apertures

Chapter 3: Face

Eye
- Inf. rectus muscle
- Lat./external rectus muscle
- Lens
- Medial/internal rectus muscle
- Optic nerve
- Sup. rectus muscle

Facial Bones
- Inf. nasal conchae or turbinates
- Lacrimal bones
- Mandible
  - Condyloid processes
  - Mentum
  - Temporomandibular joint
- Maxillary bones
  - Alveolar process/ridge
  - Frontal process
  - Hard palate
  - Palatine process
- Nasal bones
- Palatine bones
- Vomer
- Zygomatic/malar bones

Miscellaneous
- Ant. clinoids of sphenoid bone
- Body of sphenoid bone
- Compact bone
- Cribriform plate
- Crista galli
- Diploe
- Mastoid air cells
- Temporal bone

Nose
- Bony nasal septum
  - Perpendicular plate of ethmoid bone
  - Vomer
- Inf. nasal concha/turbinate
- Middle nasal concha/turbinate
- Septal cartilage
- Sup. nasal concha/turbinate

Orbit
- Inf. orbital margin
- Orbital bones
  - Ethmoid bone—lat. mass
  - Frontal bone—roof
  - Lacrimal bone
  - Maxillary bone
  - Palatine bone
  - Sphenoid bone
  - Zygomatic bone
- Sup. orbital margin

Paranasal Sinuses
- Ethmoid
- Frontal
- Maxillary
- Sphenoid

Chapter 4: Neck

Blood Vessels
Ant. communicating arteries

Ant. jugular vein, R/L

Aorta

    Ascending aorta

    Descending aorta

Common carotid artery, R/L

External carotid artery, R/L

External jugular vein, R/L

Internal carotid artery, R/L

    Ant. cerebral arteries

    Middle cerebral arteries

Internal jugular vein, R/L

Pulmonary trunk

    Pulmonary artery, R/L

R brachiocephalic artery

Subclavian artery, R/L

Vertebral artery, R/L

    Basilar artery

        Post. cerebral arteries

Esophagus

Hyoid Bone

Larynx
Arytenoids

Corniculates

Cricoid cartilage

Cuneiforms

Epiglottis

Thyroid cartilage

Miscellaneous
Mandible

Muscles
Erector spinae

Longus capitis

Longus colli

Platysma

Scalene muscles (ant., middle, post.)

Sternocleidomastoid (SCM)

Sternohyoid/sternothyroid

Pharynx
Laryngopharynx

Salivary Glands
Parotid

Sublingual

Submandibular

Thyroid Gland

Trachea
Tracheal cartilage

Chapter 5: Thorax

Blood Vessels

Aorta
- Ascending aorta
- Arch of aorta
  - L common carotid artery
  - L subclavian artery
  - R brachiocephalic artery
    - R common carotid artery
    - R subclavian artery
- Descending aorta
  - Abdominal
  - Thoracic

Inferior vena cava (IVC)
Pulmonary trunk
- Pulmonary arteries, R/L
Pulmonary veins, R/L
Superior vena cava (SVC)
- Azygos vein
  - Azygos arch
    - Hemiazygos vein
  - Brachiocephalic vein, R/L

Clavicle

Acromial end
Sternal end

Esophagus

Heart

Apex
Base
Bicuspid/mitral valve
Chambers
- Atrium, R/L
- Ventricle, R/L

Interatrial septum
Interventricular septum
Pericardium
Tricuspid valve

Liver

Lungs

Apex
Base
Cardiac notch
Hilum
Root of the lung

Miscellaneous

Margin of mediastinum

Muscles

Ant.
- Pectoralis major
- Pectoralis minor
- Subclavius

Lat.
- Serratus ant.

Post.
- Erector spinae
- Latissimus dorsi
- Levator scapulae
- Rhomboid major
- Rhomboid minor
- Serratus posterior inf.
- Serratus posterior sup.
- Splenius capitis
- Splenius colli
- Trapezius

| Muscles of the thorax |
| Diaphragm |
| Intercostal (external, internal) |

Ribs

| Head |
| Tubercle |

Sternum

| Body/gladiolus |
| Jugular/suprasternal notch |

| Manubrium |
| Sternal angle |
| Sternoclavicular/SC joint |
| Xiphoid/ensiform process |

Thymus

Trachea

| Carina |
| Primary bronchus, R/L |
| Secondary bronchi, R/L |

Chapter 6: Abdomen

Adrenal Or Suprarenal, R/L

Blood Vessels
Azygos vein
Common iliac artery, R/L
Descending aorta (abdominal, thoracic)
  Celiac axis/artery/trunk
    Common hepatic artery
    L gastric artery
    Splenic artery
  Inf. mesenteric artery (IMA)
  Renal artery, R/L
  Sup. mesenteric artery (SMA)
Hemiazygos vein
Inferior vena cava (IVC)
  Hepatic veins
    Hepatic vein, R/L
    Middle hepatic vein
  Renal vein, R/L
Portal vein
  Inf. mesenteric vein (IMV)
  L gastric vein
  Splenic vein
  Sup. mesenteric vein (SMV)

Esophagus
Cardiac orifice
Esophagogastric junction

Gallbladder

Heart
Interventricular septum
Pericardium
Ventricle, R/L

Intestines
Large
  Anus
  Ascending colon
  Cecum
  Descending colon
  Hepatic flexure
  Ileocecal valve
  Rectum
  Sigmoid colon
  Splenic flexure
  Transverse colon
  Vermiform appendix/appendix
Small
  Duodenum
  Ileum
  Jejunum

Liver
Falciform ligament
L lobe
Ligamentum teres/round ligament
Ligamentum venosum
Longitudinal fissure
Porta hepatis
R lobe
  Caudate lobe
  Quadrate lobe
Umbilical notch

Miscellaneous
Iliac crest
Lung
Rib

Spinal canal

Spinal cord

Sternum

Umbilicus

Muscles

Diaphragm

Aortic hiatus

Caval hiatus

Crus, R/L

Esophageal hiatus

Hemidiaphragm

Erector spinae

Iliacus

Intercostal

Lateral

External oblique

Internal oblique

Transversus abdominis

Psoas

Quadratus lumborum

Rectus abdominis

Linea alba

Pancreas

Body

Head

Neck

Tail

Peritoneum

Retroperitoneal space

Pararenal space (ant., post.)

Perirenal space

Spleen

Stomach

Body

Duodenum

Fundus

Greater curvature

Lesser curvature

Pylorus

Pyloric antrum

Pyloric sphincter

Urinary System

Bladder

Kidney, R/L

Cortex

Hilum

Major calyces

Medulla

Renal pelvis

Ureter, R/L

Chapter 7: Pelvis

Blood Vessels

Aorta

    Common iliac artery, R/L

    External iliac artery, R/L

    Femoral artery, R/L

    Internal iliac artery, R/L

Inferior vena cava (IVC)

    Femoral vein, R/L

    External iliac vein, R/L

    Internal iliac vein, R/L

    Common iliac vein, R/L

Female Reproductive Organs

Ovary, R/L

Uterine/fallopian tubes/oviducts

Uterus

    Cavity

    Cervix

    Fundus

Vagina

Intestines

Large

    Anus

    Ascending colon

    Cecum

    Descending colon

    Hepatic flexure

    Rectum

    Sigmoid

    Splenic flexure

    Vermiform appendix/appendix

Small

    Duodenum

    Ileum

    Jejunum

Male Reproductive Organs

Bulbourethral gland

Ductus vas deferens

Prostate gland

Scrotum

Seminal vesicle

Testis or testicles

Muscles

Erector spinae

Gluteal

    Maximus

    Medius

    Minimus

Iliacus

    Iliopsoas

Lateral

    External oblique

    Internal oblique

    Transversus abdominis

Levator ani

Obturator

    Externus

    Internus

Pectineus

Piriformis/pyriformis

Psoas

Rectus abdominis

Linea alba

Rectus femoris

Sartorius

Tensor

Pelvic Bony Structures

Coccyx

Femur

Greater trochanter

Head

Lesser trochanter

Hip/innominate bones/os coxae

Acetabulum

Ilium

Ala

Body

Crest

Greater sciatic notch

Inf. iliac spine, ant. and sup.

Sup. iliac spine, ant. and sup.

Ischium

Body

Inf. ramus

Ischial spine

Ischial tuberosity

Obturator foramen, R/L

Pubic bone

Body

Inf. ramus

Sup. ramus

Symphysis pubis

Sacroiliac joint/SI joint

Sacrum

Body

Foramina

Lateral masses

Promontory

Segment

Urinary System

Bladder

Kidney, R/L

Ureter, R/L

Urethra

Chapter 8: Vertebral Column

Atypical Vertebra

Ant. arch C1
Atlas C1
Axis C2
Bifid spinous process
Body
Intervertebral foramen
Lamina
Lat. masses
Odontoid process of C2
Pedicle
Post. arch C1
Sacrum
Spinous process
Sup. articulating facet C1
Transverse foramen
Transverse process
Vertebra prominens
Vertebral arch
Vertebral foramen

Intervertebral Disk

Annulus fibrosus
Nucleus pulposus

Ligaments

Ant. longitudinal ligament ALL
Ligamentum flava
Ligamentum nuchae
Post. longitudinal ligament PLL
Supraspinous ligament

Spinal Cord

Cauda equina
Central canal—CSF
Cervical enlargement
Conus medullaris
Lumbar enlargement

Typical Vertebra

Body
Inf. articulating process
Intervertebral foramen
Lamina
Pedicle
Spinous process
Sup. articulating process
Transverse process
Vertebral foramen
Vertebral/neural arch
Vertebral notch
Vertebral/spinal canal
Zygoapophyseal/apophyseal joint

Miscellaneous

Foramen magnum
Medulla oblongata
Occipital bone
Vertebral artery

Chapter 9: Upper Extremity

Bursae
Subacromial/subdeltoid

Carpal Bones
Capitate

Hamate

Lunate

Pisiform

Scaphoid

Trapezium

Trapezoid

Triquetrum

Clavicle
Acromial end

Humerus
Anatomic neck

Bicipital groove

Capitulum

Condyle (lat., medial)

Coronoid fossa

Epicondyle (lat., medial)

Head

Olecranon fossa

Shaft

Trochlea

Tubercle (greater, lesser)

Ligaments
Acromioclavicular ligament

Annular

Coracohumeral

Flexor retinaculum manus

Radial or medial collateral

Ulnar or lat. collateral

Miscellaneous
Acromioclavicular (AC) joint

Carpal tunnel

Labrum (ant., inf., post., sup.)

Metacarpals (1–5)

Rib

Rotator cuff

Shoulder joint

Muscles
Anconeus

Biceps brachii

Brachialis

Brachioradialis

Deltoid

Extensor

Extensor carpi radialis

Extensor carpi radialis longus

Flexor

Infraspinatus

Pectoralis

Pronator teres

Subscapularis

Supinator

Supraspinatus

Triceps

Triceps brachii

Radius
Distal radius

Head

Neck

Styloid process

Tuberosity

Scapula
Acromion
Axillary border
Coracoid process
Glenoid fossa
Neck
Spine
Styloid process

Ulna
Coronoid process
Distal ulna
Olecranon process
Radial notch
Styloid process

Chapter 10: Lower Extremity

Blood Vessels
Popliteal artery
Popliteal vein

Bursa
Prepatella
Suprapatellar

Femur
Condyle (lat., medial)
Distal femur
Fovea capitis
Greater trochanter
Head
Intercondylar fossa
Intercondylar tubercle
Intertrochanteric crest
Neck
Trochanter (greater, lesser)

Fibula
Lat. malleolus

Joints
Mortise
Subtalar
Tibiotalar

Ligaments
Ant. cruciate
Ant. talofibular
Deltoid
Iliofemoral
Interosseous talocalcaneal
Lat. collateral

Lat. patellar retinaculum
Ligamentum teres femoris
Medial collateral
Medial patellar retinaculum
Patellar
Post. cruciate
Post. talofibular
Post. tibiofibular
Spring
Tibiotalar
Transverse ligament

Miscellaneous
Articular capsule
Articular cartilage
Infrapatellar fat pad
Joint capsule
Labrum
Meniscus (lat., medial)
Sacrum
Sinus tarsi

Muscles
Achilles tendon of gastrocnemius and
  soleus muscles
Adductor
Adductor brevis
Adductor longus
Adductor magnus
Biceps femoris
Extensor digitorum longus
Extensor hallucis longus
Flexor digitorum longus
Flexor hallucis longus

Gastrocnemius
Lat. head
Medial head
Gemellus
Gluteal
Maximus
Medius
Minimus
Gracilis
Iliacus
Iliopsoas
Obturator
Externus
Internus
Pectineus
Peroneus brevis
Peroneus longus
Peroneus tertius
Piriformis
Plantaris
Popliteus
Psoas
Quadratus femoris
Quadriceps
Rectus femoris
Sartorius
Semimembranosus
Semitendinosus
Superior gemellus
Tensor
Tibialis ant.
Tibialis post.
Vastus intermedius muscle
Vastus lateralis
Vastus medialis

Patella
Apex
Base

Pelvic Girdle
Acetabulum
Fossa
Roof
Ilium
Body
Ischium
Spine
Tuberosity
Pubis
Body
Ramus (inf., sup.)
Symphysis pubis -

Tarsal Bones
Calcaneus
Sustentaculum tali
Cuboid
Cuneiform
First/medial
Second/intermediate
Third/lat.
Navicular
Talus
Head
Lat. process
Post. process
Trochlea

Tibia
Condyle (lat., medial)
Intercondylar eminence
Intercondylar tubercle
Medial malleolus
Proximal tibia
Tibial plateau